Strategies for Healthcare Education
HOW TO TEACH IN THE 21ST CENTURY

Strategies for Healthcare Education

HOW TO TEACH IN THE 21ST CENTURY

Edited by

JAN WOODHOUSE

MEd, PGDE, BN (Hons), DipN, RGN, OND, FETC

Senior Lecturer
School of Health & Social Care
University of Chester

Foreword by

DOROTHY MARRISS

Deputy Vice Chancellor
University of Chester

Radcliffe Publishing
Oxford • Seattle

Radcliffe Publishing Ltd
18 Marcham Road
Abingdon
Oxon OX14 1AA
United Kingdom

www.radcliffe-oxford.com
Electronic catalogue and worldwide online ordering facility.

British Library Cataloguing in Publication Data

A catalogue record for this book is available from the British Library.

ISBN-10: 1 84619 006 1
ISBN-13: 978 1 84619 006 3

Typeset by Egan Reid Ltd, Auckland, New Zealand
Printed and bound by Biddles Ltd, King's Lynn, Norfolk, UK

Contents

Foreword

This book gives the reader an immensely readable account of the move that healthcare education has made into the twenty-first century.

As recently as 20 years ago healthcare education was very much about didactic 'old-style' learning – 'chalk and talk', limited learning resources, set textbooks and teachers focusing on the 'how' of care delivery. Theory was not at a deep enough level to explain fully the 'why' of care delivery. Practitioners and teachers resisted challenge and questioning from students, who then took on a subservient role, working and learning in a highly disciplined manner.

The move from a syllabus of training that detailed concise statements in relation to learning to a curriculum for education that emphasises learning strategy and outcomes is a fairly recent development in education planning. Now the teacher is a facilitator of learning, with the expertise to create a stimulating learning environment.

The strategies outlined in this book will help the teacher to support professional standards by facilitating the learning of healthcare students through experiential approaches. The strategies that are described are covered from a theoretical point of view as well as from an experiential perspective. The contributors have utilised reflection and experience and considered the advantages and disadvantages of each strategy, coming up with a summary and suggestions for its use. Evidence-based care is facilitated by enabling healthcare students to learn experientially to develop reflective skills and make connections between theory and practice, thereby gaining the competence to take the initiative.

This book is primarily aimed at the new teacher in healthcare education, with a focus on the multi-professional dimension. I highly recommend it both as a rich source of education development for the new teacher and as a refresher for the more experienced teacher.

Dorothy Marriss
Deputy Vice Chancellor
University of Chester
November 2006

Preface

A couple of years ago my colleagues and I were undertaking the Postgraduate Diploma in Education for Nurses and Midwives. The course gave the theoretical background to what we had already encountered as teachers in practice and in higher education. As part of the course we were invited to explore the teaching strategies that we used.

Researching these was not easy, as books on educational topics tended to make only passing reference to the various strategies available. Few made reference to the suitability of different strategies for the particular topics that we encounter in healthcare education. The journals were sometimes more fruitful, and on occasion there was actual research to validate one method over another. Even so, we had to cast our net widely and we drew articles from a variety of disciplines, including general education, management, the aviation industry, drama and language teaching. For some strategies the searches yielded little, indicating that they have not been fully debated because they are relatively new.

By the time we reached the end of the course we had amassed a fine collection of research between us, and there the story could have ended. The knowledge that we had gained could have stayed with us, the research findings gathering dust on a shelf or, worse still, shredded for recycling. Meanwhile the students who followed in our footsteps would start the search all over again, with the spectre of a similar ending to their research. However, as we completed our studies, the opportunity arose to compile a book – the one that now lies in front of you. It seemed eminently sensible to collate our research findings and pass on the knowledge that we had gained through our practice and enquiries to others who may be new to using different teaching strategies.

Obviously, as my colleagues and I are all healthcare professionals, we have focused on those topics that are taught in our discipline. However, the strategies are applicable to many disciplines. It all depends on what is being taught, which domain is being targeted, the learning styles of the student and the teaching style of the tutor. As we have 'borrowed' knowledge from elsewhere during the course of our research, this book aims to give back to other disciplines, too. For although the title of the book mentions teaching strategies for healthcare education, it would be just as useful for someone starting in general education, management, the aviation industry, drama or language teaching. The important thing is to share knowledge and not let it gather dust on the shelf, either physically or metaphorically. The aim of this book is to promote evidence-based teaching – a concept heralded by the twenty-first century. We hope that it will be of use to both neophyte and experienced teachers.

Jan Woodhouse
November 2006

List of contributors

Jan Gidman BSc (Hons), MEd, RGN, ONC
Head of Practice Learning, School of Health & Social Care, University of Chester

Steve Hardman BSc (Hons), PGCHE, Dip N, RGN
Senior Lecturer in Adult Nursing Studies, School of Health & Social Care, University of Chester

Adam Keen MSc, MEd, Dip HE, RN
Senior Lecturer in Adult Nursing Studies, School of Health & Social Care, University of Chester

Jean Mannix BSc (Hons), Nurse Prescriber, RGN
Community Practice Teacher/Senior Lecturer in Practice Learning, School of Health & Social Care, University of Chester

Gill Murphy BA (Hons), MA, PGDE, RMN
Senior Lecturer in Mental Health Studies, School of Health & Social Care, University of Chester

Sue Padmore BA (Hons), RN, RM
Senior Lecturer in Adult Nursing Studies, School of Health & Social Care, University of Chester

Debbie Robertson BSc (Hons), PhD, RGN
Senior Lecturer in Non-Medical Prescribing, School of Health & Social Care, University of Chester

Liz Sweet MSc, PGDip Nursing, BN, RNT, HV Cert, NDN Cert, SRN
Senior Lecturer, Department of Work Related Studies, School of Business and Law, University of Chester

Jan Woodhouse BN (Hons), MEd, PGDE, Dip N, RGN, OND, FETC
Senior Lecturer in Adult Nursing Studies/Programme Leader for MSc in Advanced Practice, School of Health & Social Care, University of Chester

Acknowledgements

Thanks are due first to Val Thornes, Programme Leader for the Masters degree in Education for Nurses and Midwives, without whom the whole topic of investigating teaching strategies in healthcare education would not have arisen.

Secondly, we wish to thank the contributors and others at the School of Health & Social Care, University of Chester, who gave the writing of this book their unwavering support.

Thirdly, we would like to thank the partners and colleagues of all the contributors for providing support in terms of time, proofreading, helpful suggestions and just 'being there.'

Finally, thanks are due to two pre-registration nursing students, Angela Roberts and Amy Chrimes, who gave up their time to help with the Vancouver style of referencing.

CHAPTER 1

Introduction: from the twentieth to the twenty-first century

Jan Woodhouse

The journey

In order to consider how to teach in the twenty-first century, it is perhaps wise to look back at the twentieth century both to see where we have come from and to understand the changes in approaches to education. Turning back the clock to the early 1900s would lead us into the classroom setting, where the main resources were chalk and blackboards. There was a limited range of books available, and those that did exist were expensive and contained only a limited amount of graphic material. It is hardly surprising that the main teaching strategy was the lecture – in which notes

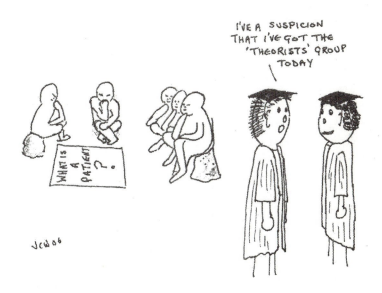

were dictated, diagrams were copied from the blackboard and the knowledge base was often based on opinion rather than on research.

With these scarce resources it is hardly surprising that the educational ideology that predominated was the acquisition of knowledge by the process of memorising information. Hence the teaching strategies used were repetition, rote learning and the use of mnemonics. Assessment of learning involved testing of the memory by means of oral, written and/or practical examinations. Often the learning that took place was purely for the purpose of passing examinations and bore no context to the work environment in which the students would later find themselves.

Healthcare education in the early 1900s had two strands, namely medical education based in universities, and unregulated schools of nursing based in local hospitals. The 'medical model' was a method of teaching in which history taking, signs and symptoms, diagnosis and treatment formed the basis of education for doctors and nurses alike. Doctors were taught more anatomy and physiology, dissection, chemistry, microbiology and examination skills, whereas nurses were taught cookery for the sick, along with bathing and bandaging techniques. By today's standards the knowledge base for both professions was small. The education received was considered sufficient to last a lifetime and was very broad, so that an individual could step into any situation, whether in hospital or in the community, and be served by that education. The post that an individual obtained was theirs for life, so any additional knowledge gained was learned through experience.

As the twentieth century progressed, emerging healthcare professions became established, including radiologists, pharmacists, physiotherapists, occupational therapists, speech and language therapists, psychologists and nutritionists, to name just a few, as well as specialisms within the disciplines.

As our knowledge base increases so does the demand for specialism, because we can no longer expect to know everything about healthcare as we might have done 100 years ago. In the twenty-first century we are aware that learning is a lifelong process, and in order to keep up with the rapidly expanding knowledge base we have to participate in continuing professional development. It is no longer acceptable to base our practice on the opinion of one individual – we must use evidence to support the care that we deliver. We no longer have jobs for life – organisations are always seeking new ways to deliver value-for-money services, which means that an individual may have to change their practice by acquiring new skills or working in a different fashion. The ideology of transferable skills comes to the fore. Alongside it, the notion of working as a team towards a shared goal is enhanced by inter-professional learning.

The concept of the professions learning together has been enhanced by several higher education institutions (HEIs) which have curricula that bring student doctors, nurses, physiotherapists and others together in a way that would not have been dreamed of even 50 years ago.

The twentieth century also saw a technological revolution as a result of the development of photography, cinematography, sound-recording equipment, radio, television, telephone, video, computers, the Internet and digital imagery. One by one, these marvels have found their way into the classroom until we have reached the stage of the 'virtual classroom', where teachers and students meet in cyberspace. This means that our students' needs now differ from those previously encountered. There may be residues of the dependent relationship that existed a century ago, but the likelihood is that self-directed learning will increasingly predominate for the student. Indeed it is a quality that is currently encouraged in students and is supported by Knowles' concept of andragogy.[1]

This brings us to another aspect of change. Our knowledge of learning and teaching has expanded exponentially, so the following sections of this chapter address those aspects that any teacher who is new to the profession needs to consider before they step in front of their students.

The work of the theorists

It was in the early twentieth century that interest in how learning takes place became the subject of research. A plethora of scientists have postulated theories and researched on this topic, and although this book cannot cover them all, it is worth mentioning those who do appear frequently in the healthcare literature, and those who are included in subsequent chapters of this book. Some of the theorists have been grouped under schools of thought and are known as *behaviourists, cognitivists* and *humanists*.[2]

- *Behaviourists.* The names that get a mention in this category include Thorndike (learning curve), Pavlov (stimulus/response and classical conditioning) and Skinner (the importance of pleasurable rewards as reinforcers). These ideas have been developed, and one could include Berne, who proposed transactional analysis theory and considers that 'positive' and 'negative' strokes to the self-esteem play an important part in our learning.
- *Cognitivists.* One of the early theorists in this category is Piaget, who considered that we process information as a schema. He recognised that different types of learning takes place as we develop from infancy to adulthood. Another theorist in this school is Gagné, who identified different types of learning, also related to age, such as verbal association and problem solving. One could also include Dreyfus and Benner here, as their work is particularly relevant to the field of healthcare education. They acknowledge that in terms of skills acquisition a learner moves from being a novice to being a potential expert.
- *Humanists.* In this category, which takes the stance that we are individualistic in our learning, the names of Maslow (motivational hierarchy of needs), Bandura (social learning theory and role modelling) and Rogers (self-directed learning and unconditional positive regard) are prominent. These theorists remind us that our learners are people – who learn from each other, and have different driving forces and life problems.

There is a further school of thought known as *constructivism*,[3] according to which knowledge itself is a constructed entity that is reliant on individual interpretation. For example, ask someone to define 'pain' and you will get a raft of different answers.

Perhaps it is time, though, to add another school, as it is such a prevalent notion in the healthcare literature, namely *reflectionism*.

■ *Reflectionists.* The names that feature in this school are Dewey[4] (interaction, reflection and experience), Lewin[5] (groups, experiential learning and action research), Kolb[1] (the learning cycle) and Schön (reflecting in action and reflecting on action, and double loop learning).[6] All of these theorists pay heed to what goes on inside an individual's head – their thinking – and give due regard to the idea that we can use this to identify learning. Not only that, but we can start to think in a different way – a reflective way.

Finally, there are some theorists who help us to consider what we teach and who we teach. What we teach has been considered by Bloom,[7] utilising a taxonomy divided into three domains – cognitive, affective and psychomotor. Within each of these domains the student can demonstrate progression using the taxonomy. Similarly, Steinaker and Bell[8] have produced a taxonomy of experiential learning by identifying the stages of exposure, participation, identification, internalisation and dissemination. These taxonomies help the teacher to consider the levels of learning attained by the student and give direction to future goals.

With regard to 'who we teach', Knowles considers the notion of andragogy (adult and self-directed learners) versus pedagogy (learners who rely on being led).[1] The hope is that the student will move from dependency (such as that experienced in primary and secondary education) to independence (as promoted in higher education). In addition, the teacher must also have an awareness of another aspect of the 'who', and give consideration to the individuality of the students that they teach. This can be achieved by the recognition, knowledge and influence of different learning styles.

Learning styles

At the beginning of the twentieth century the classification of individuals was simplistic and, for some, had the potential to do psychological damage. Students were labelled using terms such as 'clever', 'quick', 'stupid', 'daft' and 'dunce.' Everyone was taught by the same approach and there was no room for differences. Then the concept of measuring IQ came into use, and there was an objective, numerical score to either confirm or deny the labels. However, individuals realised as they went through life that the initial labels that had been given to them at school no longer held true when they were adult, and that academic achievement was within their reach. What had changed for them was that they recognised that they had learned things outside the classroom, possibly because they were 'doing' – that is, having a hands-on, practical experience.

Today we have reached the point of recognition of the individualism of learning. Educationalists now take a more constructivist view and seek to identify particular learning styles in order to enhance learning. Several models will emerge within the following chapters.

One such model is that of Kolb,[9] who considers the different processes of concrete and abstract thinking, together with experimentation and observation. This gives rise to four categories of learners, namely *divergers, convergers, assimilators* and *accommodators*. Students will have a preferred leaning towards one of the categories. For example, I am a diverger – I prefer using reflective observation and having a concrete experience over abstraction and experimentation.

Another model that is frequently referred to is that of Honey and Mumford,[1] who draw on Kolb's work, where students are categorised as *activists, pragmatists, reflectors* or *theorists*. Again I score highly on the reflective element of this model, although as I have progressed through academia, my scores on the theorist section have risen. This demonstrates that students may similarly change styles as they progress through their lifelong learning.

There are also models that consider the cognitive processes, and these are denoted by the abbreviations V-A-K[10] and VARK.[11] These letters stand for visual (V), auditory (A), reading/writing (R) and kinaesthetic (K) learners. In other words, the student has a preferred sense that is used to enhance learning. The visual learner may prefer pictures, videos, diagrams and charts, whereas the auditory learner prefers lectures and sounds. The reader/writer learner likes to do just that – read and make notes, whereas the kinaesthetic learner needs to handle items such as handouts or models.

Neurolinguistic programming (NLP)[12] also makes reference to individuals thinking in terms of pictures, sound and feeling (here 'feeling' is referred to the emotional content, not the kinaesthetic/touch aspect). However, NLP also recognises that the other senses of taste, touch and smell are associated with memories, and therefore if aspects of these are incorporated into sessions then learning may be enhanced.

Still further work considers the functional aspects of the brain. This gives rise to the notion of left brain/right brain thinking.[13] The left side of the brain is the logical side, where processes such as mathematics, organisation and problem solving take place. The right side of the brain deals with the imagination and interpersonal aspects, so communication, creativity and relationships may be processed here. These concepts have given rise to the idea that there may be gender differences in the way that we learn.

If the teacher has the time, identifying the preferred style of the individual or the group may be a useful indicator when choosing what teaching strategy to adopt. However, the more learning styles that are identified the more difficult it becomes to tailor teaching to a particular style. Consequently, the teacher has to adopt several strategies within a teaching session in order to match the variety of styles. The underlying principle that has to be acknowledged is that in each interaction between the teacher and the student the learning opportunity is maximised. Similarly, it is important to recognise that teachers also have their own preferences with regard to the way in which they teach. This brings us to the topic of teaching styles, which are referred to several times in subsequent chapters of this book, acknowledging the relationship between the quality of teaching and the quality of learning.

Teaching styles

As early as the beginning of the twentieth century, consideration was given to what makes a good teacher. One only has to turn to the realms of English literature to discover writers on the topic, such as Dickens. We can all recall a significant teacher whom we encountered during our years of education. Within this book several reflections draw on memories of school and the strategies that were used by teachers. This highlights the importance of the relationship between the student and the teacher, and the effect that it has on learning.

Even the terms that are used to describe the person who leads the learning experience reflect different styles of teaching. For example, a 'lecturer' implies that the teacher 'stands and delivers' to a group – that is, there is a one-way transmission of information, from the lecturer to the students. The term 'teacher' takes us back to primary and secondary education, where the group is a 'class' and the delivery is a 'lesson.' The word 'tutor' has a personal air and seems more appropriate for higher education, as it tends to suggest that an academic relationship forms between the tutor and the student. Another term, which has been used more recently, is 'facilitator.' This acknowledges that people learn from each other and that the role of the teacher is to encourage the sharing of knowledge. So what we call ourselves may be part of the academic debate. However, even if the title is fixed, as mine is, this does not mean that it limits the teaching style.

In the same way that learning styles have been explored, there has also been research on teaching styles. A recent concept is that of *conservative* and *progressive* teachers.[14] The conservative teacher is more likely to follow traditional ways of teaching, namely didactic delivery, lecturing, and tried and trusted methods, whereas the progressive teacher seeks different approaches, is willing to try new strategies and encourages interaction.

An alternative model is that of the four styles proposed by Gilmartin.[15] Type 1 uses a didactic style, type 2 combines a didactic method with experiential activities, type 3 favours student-centred facilitation and type 4 aims for creative approaches. These typologies are further enhanced by different methods of facilitation, which Gilmartin refers to as type X (closed) and type Y (open). The closed style is authoritarian, detached and critical, with minimal involvement of the student, whereas the open style is spontaneous, involved and committed, and responds to student-led initiatives.

The final model to be described here is that of Grasha.[16] It reflects the activity pursued by the person at the front of the class, and includes five categories, namely *expert, formal authority, personal model, facilitator* and *delegator*. The expert is concerned with the transmission of knowledge, the person with formal authority gains status from the students through knowledge and values, the personal model acts as a role model for students, the facilitator emphasises the interpersonal relationship between student and teacher, and the delegator seeks to enhance the autonomy of the students.

What these styles demonstrate is that there are different ways of being when working with students. For example, sometimes it may be an appropriate strategy to act in a conservative manner, while at other times it may be more appropriate to be a personal model. It is possible to use several different teaching styles within the time frame of a session. What is important is that the teaching style and the teaching strategy need to match up. For example, it is pointless to tell the students in an authoritarian manner that they *must* draw an object, as they will then rapidly disengage and provide reasons why they cannot do what has been asked of them, and thus the teaching strategy will fail. Similarly, if the students have been used to only receiving lectures, then if you step into the room with your facilitator hat on it is going to take time to establish a relationship with them that is strong enough to allow them to experiment with the idea.

Conclusion

Looking at the past century and the present one makes me realise just how much growth there has been in knowledge and research with regard to education. The continual development of resources and technology means that the demand for new practices is an essential component of teaching.

We are fortunate in that we can draw upon the work of the twentieth-century theorists to improve our understanding and to guide us in our practice. The realm of healthcare education is diverse – we have to acknowledge our scientific background, and at the same time the fact that we apply our knowledge to people means that we also have to have a humanistic perspective. We use knowledge of physics, chemistry, research, mathematics, psychology, sociology, anatomy, physiology, management and communication, to name but a few, in our everyday working life. This means that decision making about which teaching strategy to use for a particular topic is of central importance.

This book aims to bring some clarity to the situation. It is a journey into evidence-based teaching as it considers the strategies most frequently used in healthcare education, such as lectures, small group work, case study, problem-based learning and reflection, and highlights the advantages and disadvantages of each of them. In addition, more adventurous strategies are discussed, such as simulation, role play, storytelling, experiential learning exercises and creative activities. Newer strategies are also explored, including blended learning (a mix of face-to-face contact and e-learning) and self-directed study. Chapter 13 is completely different from the rest, as the author uses the topic of 'self-directed study' to carry out self-directed study herself! It sounds somewhat circular but, as a result of her self-monitoring, emerging themes are identified that help to explain the process of self-directed study. Finally, the book reflects on the different strategies that have been discussed and considers how they are applied in the practice setting.

We hope that this book will be useful to both new and experienced teachers in healthcare education, and that their students will benefit from experiencing a range of strategies that were not available in the twentieth century.

References

1 Reece I, Walker S. *Teaching, Training and Learning: a practical guide incorporating FENTO standards.* 5th ed. London: Business Education Publishers; 2003.

2 Woodhouse J. *Motivation towards education in post-registered nurses.* Unpublished Masters dissertation. Chester: University of Chester; 2003.

3 Department of Information Science, University of Bergen. *Constructivism;* www.uib.no/People/sinia/CSCL/web_struktur-836.htm (accessed 17 March 2004).

4 Dewey J. www.infed.org/thinkers/et-dewey.htm (accessed 30 March 2006).

5 Lewin K. www.infed.org/thinkers/et-lewin.htm (accessed 30 March 2006).

6 Schön D. www.infed.org/thinkers/et-schon.htm (accessed 30 March 2006).

7 *Bloom's Taxonomy;* www.learningandteaching.info/learning/bloomtax.htm (accessed 30 March 2006).

8 Mattern JL. Developing a well-worn path between classroom and workplace through managed experiential learning. *North Dakota J Speech & Theatre Assoc* [online journal]. 2003; **6**.

9 Wilson JT. *Understanding Learning Styles: implications for design education in the university;* www.arts.ac.uk/docs/cltad_202wilson.pdf (accessed 30 March 2006).

10 Putintseva T. The importance of learning styles in ESL/EFL. *Internet TESL J.* 2006; **12**; http://iteslj.org/Articles/Putintseva-LearningStyles.html (accessed 30 March 2006).

11 *VARK – a guide to learning styles;* www.vark-learn.com/english/index.asp (accessed 30 March 2006).

12 O'Connor J, Seymour J. *Introducing Neuro-Linguistic Programming.* San Francisco, CA: Thorsons; 1990.

13 Jensen E. *Brain-Based Learning.* Del Mar, CA: Turning Point Publications; 1996.

14 Robins L, Greenwood J. Groups and group work in public administration. *Public Admin.* 2000; **78**: 957–65.

15 Gilmartin J. Teachers' understanding of facilitation styles with student nurses. *Int J Nurs Stud.* 2001; **38**: 481–8.

16 Center for Instruction, Research & Technology, Indiana State University. *Grasha's Five Teaching Styles;* www.indstate.edu/ctl/styles/5styles.html (accessed 30 March 2006).

CHAPTER 2

The 'dreaded' lecture

Gill Murphy

Introduction and reflection

When I hear the term 'lecture', it automatically takes me back some years to my pre-registration nursing programme, when a class of around 200 students sat in a huge lecture theatre. Some were attempting to listen intensely despite the sound of sweet wrappers behind them, while others were dozing in the dimmed light. Some students arrived late, and indeed some chose the easy way out and headed for the exit door after just 20 minutes. Regardless of all of the interruptions, the lecturer continued with his lesson plan, determined that a few college kids would not disturb his session. His voice increased in volume a little, but seemingly with very little effect. I now

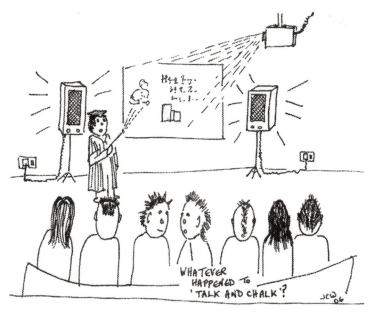

WHATEVER HAPPENED TO 'TALK AND CHALK'?

confess, some years later, that while I sat and endured the countless boring lectures, I have no recollection whatsoever of their actual content. There were times when I admired the hair of the young girl in front of me, or I wrote a message to the guy sitting a few seats away from me, who I had fancied for ages, and this seemed like the perfect opportunity to make a move: *'What do you think of this? Rubbish, isn't it?'*

Does any of this sound familiar to you? I could continue with similar stories and reflections. In contrast, however, I can recall the actual conversations, the layout of the room and the people I sat next to in one session when the tutor appeared, alone, without an army of teaching resources. He entered the room and the show began. He facilitated group discussion, applied the ethical principles to sex and the group laughed, smiled and joked. I remember thinking at the time *'how inappropriate'*, but I had learned and absorbed the teaching material, and even today I feel able to relate it to clinical nursing practice. The difference between the two approaches seems to be the audience participation. One delivers *to* the audience and the other *with* the audience.

Some years later, after a varied clinical nursing career, I commenced my role within higher education health and social care delivery. You may ask which teaching methods and strategies I used. Well, as a new educator I succumbed to the safety of the 'dreaded' lecture. I appeared in front of the class armed with notes, handouts and a rigid lecture plan. I thought I might look daft if the students asked me something I didn't know. With limited confidence with regard to actual teaching, I would not be disturbed. The session followed one agenda – mine. I had maintained the tradition of higher education. It does seem surprising (even to me) that I utilised this method on the whole during my early days in education. However, when you feel at your most vulnerable, you stick to what you know. I knew I could deliver in relative safety. Here is a brief summary of one such session.

I was undertaking a session with 35 third-year, mental health nursing students on the assessment and care of individuals with personality disorder. Initially the students were asked to note any comments they had heard in clinical practice with regard to individuals with personality disorder. It has been acknowledged that many health and social care professionals feel ill equipped to work with patients with personality disorder.[1] Indeed some health professionals stereotype and label individuals with personality disorders with negative emotion. Comments by clinical staff such as 'the patients psychiatrists dislike' and 'abusers' support this view.[2] This attitude was reflected by additional remarks that students had heard from practice staff. Many of their views were very negative and condescending. The students were subsequently asked to note down their own thoughts reflecting the direct contact that they had had in clinical practice with people with personality disorder. Interestingly, all of the students' comments mirrored those to which they had been exposed in practice.

This is not too surprising, given the social learning theory proposed by Bandura.[3] This theory suggests that the observation and modelling of professional behaviours and attitudes promote learning. Further research by Quinn,[4] and later Castledine,[5] has reinforced the power of observation as a learning approach, and the influence of the clinical nursing environment. By way of example, Quinn[4] cites a study conducted by Kramer in 1972 in which the learning of professional attitudes by students was examined by observation of the nurse–patient interactions.

One can therefore see the relevance of using a teaching strategy that would allow the exploration of both cognitive and affective domains of learning. The use of the 'lecture' in this particular situation was helpful for passing on to the students formal information about the development of personality disorder and the international classification processes. I felt confident that all of the students had a similar level of understanding. However, the use of a lecture style in isolation did not allow facilitation of the students' frustration caused by working with people with personality disorder. One particular student questioned how she could work with a person who had harmed a child as a result of issues associated with personality disorder. Although the lecture approach did allow some learning about the possible causative factors involved, I remain doubtful whether I was able to challenge much of the pre-existing negative affective learning with the lecture style of delivery alone.

Definition

It seems somewhat difficult to provide a rigid definition of the term 'lecture.' Similarly, although the concept of 'lecturer practitioner' seems to be utilised frequently in health and social care, there also appears to be some uncertainty with regard to a clear definition.[6] One simplistic definition is 'to talk on a particular subject or read to an audience.'[7] Educational texts support this principle, confirming that a lecture involves one-way communication from a 'teacher' to a 'student.'[8] The notion of a professional in front of a group of novices appears to have been standard practice for some time. It seems that the former would take charge of the learning, while the latter passively observed.

However, more recently the concept of the 'lecture' has been challenged. Studies have compared teaching and learning outcomes with alternative teaching methods. The value and role of experiential learning and personal reflection have been reinforced.[9–11] Interestingly, both of these concepts advocate the active participation of the student in their learning, with the lecturer taking the role of 'back-seat driver.' However, despite this, the notion of the lecture does appear to be surviving when it is accompanied by innovation with regard to the methods of delivery. The concept of the 'lecture' is now being incorporated into the e-learning forum. One example of this has been offered by Wofford and colleagues,[12] who have piloted the use of a computer-based lecture. They suggest that it can target large groups of people, but with increased flexibility as individual students can assess the material on a continual basis. In addition, the computer-based lecture is able to offer greater opportunities for student interaction with the materials, which is thought to be of benefit in ensuring deep learning.

The advantages of 'lecturing'

The use of the lecture as a formal, structured, tutor-led session does allow for the transfer of information to students.[4,13,14] The format allows the development of the cognitive domain of learning. In the example I have given, the lecture style was extremely useful for ensuring that all students had a central understanding of the development of personality theories, international classifications, national policies and treatment regimes. I was able to establish the underpinning cognitive frameworks, which could be further developed with additional teaching methods. Furthermore, the use of a formalised lecture is critical in professional education where there are prescriptive guidelines from the governing bodies, such as the Nursing and Midwifery Council, with regard to the knowledge base required prior to registration and qualification.

Interestingly, Brookfield[14] highlights the fact that the use of the lecture as a teaching strategy can allow the tutor to offer moral understanding and boundaries within the professional context. The lecture design allowed me, as the lecturer, to use the acceptable terminologies which are preferred within the health and social fields. In trying to promote the work of the National Institute for Mental Health in England (NIMHE),[1] which aims to recognise the stigmas associated with people with personality disorder, one can accept that the reaffirming of professional boundaries seemed to be a priority. Furthermore, given that the students who attended the session may have had little intrinsic motivation to learn about the subject, due to the negative attitudes that they might have encountered within the clinical environment,[2] it was important to consider methods of generating interest.

Therefore it could be argued that the use of the lecture, with intermittent examples of my own positive clinical practice experiences, could increase students' intrinsic motivation. Obviously in clinical health and social care practice there are associations between practitioner motivation and quality of care. Reece and Walker[8] acknowledge that intrinsic motivation is often associated with deep learning. However, this must be examined with reference to the work of Brookfield,[14] who highlights the fact that a lecture style of delivery can be utilised to inspire students and generate in them a passion for an issue hitherto relatively unknown to them. Certainly the student feedback about the session would reflect something of this. Several students made comments during the evaluation of the session that this was the first time they had encountered any positive opinions or attitudes about caring for individuals diagnosed with personality disorder.

In a culture of increasingly multi-disciplinary health and social care learning within higher educational environments, a lecture style of delivery ensures that all of the content can be tailored to ensure that it is relevant to all multi-professional needs.

The disadvantages of 'lecturing'

The concept of reflection within health and social care education helps to forge links between theory and clinical practice. Its use is widely accepted within the health-related literature.[15,17-24] Nicklin and Kenworthy[15] have referred to Schön's writings on the notion of reflection during and after action. However, some authors have commented on the difficulties associated with reflection in action, especially for learners.[18,19] Given this, it seems appropriate that professional education enhances the skill of 'after-action reflection' on a continual basis, although one must question how effective a lecture can be in meeting this end. As previously mentioned, lectures are tutor-led and thus limit the voluntary involvement of the student group. Several students in the group that was studying the assessment and care of individuals with personality disorder highlighted high levels of emotion about incidents with which they had been involved. A lecture approach in isolation would not allow consideration of these issues, and would therefore limit the affective learning and attitudinal change. Furthermore, one could conclude that the students were passive in the learning process[25] and this particular teaching style does not enhance the andragogical and deep experience of learning. Oliver and Endersby[26] have highlighted the fact that lectures are associated with a limited opportunity for student feedback, thus allowing a 'pedagogical and didactic' approach to develop. This appears to be in conflict with the role of the teacher. Kelly[27] argues that the role should demonstrate a distinctive sharing but not domination of tutor understanding, emotions and past professional experiences. Furthermore, Clarke[28] suggests that the role of higher education should be to stimulate questioning and scrutiny by the student, not to promote tutor-generated ideas.

Health and social care education must incorporate practical skills and psychomotor learning in addition to cognitive and affective learning domains. This has certainly been acknowledged in the nurse education curriculum, *Making a Difference.*[29] Yet the lecture does not allow the development and feedback of an individual student's clinical practice skills. One could envisage that students' assessment and questioning skills could be enhanced by the use of alternative teaching styles, such as role play.

Research presented by Crowley[30] offers an alternative teaching strategy, which would facilitate the verbalisation of emotions generated by student experiences within the clinical environment. Crowley promotes the concept of 'therapeutic teaching', which has been utilised with student midwives. The strategy involves group discussions to increase awareness of the nature of the help that an individual may require. In addition, students are able to observe the skills of counselling and communication employed by the teacher. Students offer their personal and professional experiences of the issue in question – for example, bereavement. Crowley[30] acknowledges that students must be receptive to sharing of their emotions within a group situation. However, she does not elaborate on the emotional support that students may require after or outside the group exercise.

One could foresee that if a student felt emotionally vulnerable within the group or the group experience generated a very strong or long-lasting negative response, the student's motivation for future learning within the group, the subject and the strategy used might be affected. Furthermore, students may reappraise their past learning and re-contextualise it within a negative framework.[19] One would hope that this would be an infrequent occurrence, given the studies described by Davies[31] which claim that peer group support is ordinarily a factor that facilitates the professional socialisation of individual students.

Oliver and Endersby[26] reinforce the idea that tutors will naturally offer the teaching styles and strategies that they feel most comfortable and confident delivering.

The literature teems with articles highlighting the relevance of student learning styles when planning sessions, to ensure that different learning styles are addressed by a variety of teaching approaches.[4,13,14,26,29,32–36] Reece and Walker[8] acknowledge four main learning styles, namely 'visual/verbal, visual/non-verbal, tactile/kinaesthetic and auditory/verbal.' Each describes the most appropriate format for delivery of information in order to achieve optimum learning by the individual. It could be concluded that lectures are more suited to 'auditory/verbal' learners than to students with a 'visual/non-verbal' learning style.

One could argue that this may have many implications for both the quality and the quantity of learning for students with specific learning needs. For example, a student with hearing disturbances may experience some barriers to deep learning during a session that utilises the lecture style in isolation. A person who has been diagnosed with dyslexia may be excluded from the real benefit of learning, due to their impaired capability and speed of absorbing and processing information. Furthermore, one can predict that an individual who may be experiencing any level of depressive symptoms, or mental ill health such as schizophrenia, may be challenged by the level of cognitive functioning that is required to allow full absorption of the information presented by the lecturing style.[36] Given the work that has been done on the issues of social inclusion for all and the current widening participation agendas, this situation is unacceptable within higher education institutions.[37,38]

Summary

The concept of the lecture has evoked and continues to generate debate. Once seen as the principal teaching method for many, lectures are now being offered in different formats. Lecturers are combining the use of a lecture with other teaching resources – for example, computers. A lecture can be a very successful method of presenting factual information to a large group of people. However, it is advantageous to ensure that multiple teaching methods are employed in each session in order to ensure that the learning styles and individual needs of all students are catered for.

- ❏ Lectures enable the transfer of large amounts of information from tutor to students, especially in settings where there are high numbers of students.
- ❏ The use of the lecture ensures that the student receives accurate information when professional education requires prescribed knowledge frameworks for registration.
- ❏ Lectures can be helpful to those who are new to the higher education environment, as they offer a sense of safety under the direction of the session.
- ❏ Lectures can hinder learning by individuals with specific learning difficulties and some people with mental health problems.

□ It is questionable whether the use of lectures really enhances deep learning and addresses the gaps between theory and practice in health and social care education.

□ Lectures can be a successful teaching method in all aspects of health and social care education, if they are combined with alternative methods to promote affective and psychomotor learning.

References

1 National Institute for Mental Health in England. *Personality Disorder: no longer a diagnosis of exclusion. Policy implementation guidance for the development of services for people with personality disorder.* London: National Institute for Mental Health in England; 2003.

2 Tredget JE. The aetiology, presentation and treatment of personality disorders. *J Psychiatry Ment Health Nurs.* 2001; **8**: 347–62.

3 Bandura A. *Social Learning Theory;* http://tip.psychology.org/bandura.html (accessed 17 April 2004).

4 Quinn FM. *Principles and Practice of Nurse Education.* 4th ed. Cheltenham: Stanley Thornes (Publishers) Ltd; 2000.

5 Castledine G. Nurse education: is it becoming too academic? *Br J Nurs.* 2000; **12**: 994.

6 Elcock K. Lecturer practitioner: a concept analysis. *J Adv Nurs.* 1998; **28**: 1092–8.

7 Hanks P *et al. The Collins Paperback English Dictionary.* Glasgow: HarperCollins; 1990.

8 Reece I, Walker S. *Teaching, Training and Learning: a practical approach incorporating FENTO standards.* 5th ed. Sunderland: Business Education Publishers Ltd; 2003.

9 Smith A. Learning about reflection. *J Adv Learn.* 1998; **28**: 891–8.

10 Eraut M. Learning contexts (editorial). *Learn Health Soc Care.* 2006; **5**: 1–8.

11 Dewar BJ, Walker E. Experiential learning: issues for supervision. *J Adv Nurs.* 1999; **30**: 1459–67.

12 Wofford M, Spickard A, Wofford J. The computer-based lecture. *J Gen Intern Med.* 2001; **16**: 464–72.

13 Reed J, Proctor S. *Nurse Education: a reflective approach.* London: Edward Arnold; 1993.

14 Brookfield SD. *The Skillful Teacher.* San Francisco, CA: Jossey-Bass; 1990.

15 Nicklin P, Kenworthy N. *Teaching and Assessing in Nursing Practice.* 2nd ed. London: Scutari Press; 1995.

16 Durgahee T. *Reflective Practice: linking theory and practice in palliative care nursing;* www.internurse.com/cgi-bin/go.pl/library/article?uid (accessed 30 March 2004).

17 Vaughan B. The lecturer practitioner forum: position paper on the future of teachers. *Br J Community Nurs.* 1996; **1**: 132–3.

18 Castledine G. How to improve the morale of nursing students. *Br J Nurs.* 1998; **7**: 290.

19 Chambers N. Close encounters: the use of critical reflective analysis as an evaluation tool in teaching and learning. *J Adv Nurs.* 1999; **29**: 950–60.

20 Jackson KB. The role of the lecturer/practitioner in midwifery. *Br J Midwifery.* 1999; **7**: 363–6.

21 Eaton A. Assessing learning needs. In: Hinchliff S, editor. *The Practitioner as Teacher.* 2nd ed. London: Bailliere Tindall; 1999.

22 Gilmartin J. Teachers' understanding of facilitation styles with student nurses. *Int J Nurs Stud.* 2000; **38:** 481–8.

23 Fawcett TN, Jarvis A. Debate continues over all graduate profession (correspondence). *Br J Nurs.* 2003; **12:** 9.

24 Burnard P. Improving through reflection. *J District Nursing.* 1991; **May:** 10–12.

25 Dave RH, Armstrong RJ. *Developing and Writing Behavioral Objectives.* Tucson, AZ: Educational Innovators Press; 1970.

26 Oliver R, Endersby C. *Teaching and Assessing Nurses: a handbook for preceptors.* London: Baillière Tindall; 2000.

27 Kelly C. *Experiential Learning (C. Rogers)*; http://tip.psychology.org/rogers.html (accessed 12 November 2002).

28 Clarke L. Nurse education: why Socrates would disapprove. *Nurs Standard.* 2003; **17:** 36–7.

29 Department of Health. *Making a Difference. Strengthening the nursing, midwifery and health visiting contribution to health and healthcare.* London: Department of Health; 1999.

30 Crowley J. Therapeutic teaching and the education of student midwives. *Br J Midwifery.* 1997; **5:** 159–62.

31 Davies BD. How nurses learn and how to improve the learning environment. *Nurs Educ Today.* 1990; **10:** 405–9.

32 Kelly C. *David Kolb: the theory of experiential learning and ESL*; http://iteslij.org/Articles/Kelly-Experiential/ (accessed 12 November 2002).

33 Cantor JA. *Experiential Learning in Higher Education: linking classroom and community*; www.ntlf.com/html/lib/bib/95-7dig.htm (accessed 12 November 2002).

34 Atherton JS. *Tacit Knowledge and Implicit Learning*; www.dmu.ac.uk/-jamesa/learning/tacit.htm (accessed 1 April 2004).

35 Shailer B. *Clinical Electives: the challenge and benefits of student choice*; www.internurse.com/cgi-bin/go.pl/library/article (accessed 30 March 2004).

36 Mayer RE. *Thinking, Problem Solving, Cognition.* 2nd ed. New York: WH Freeman and Company; 1992.

37 Repper J, Perkins R. *Social Inclusion and Recovery: a model for mental health practice.* London: Baillière Tindall; 2003.

38 Higher Education Funding Council for England. *Higher Education Funding Council for England Strategic Plan 2003 – August 2005*; www.hefce.ac.uk/pubs/hefce/2005/05_16/05_16.doc (accessed 21 March 2006).

CHAPTER 3

Small group learning: greater than the sum of its parts?

Adam Keen

Introduction

Groups are a prominent feature within our society.[1] Consequently, it is unsurprising to find that group structures represent a major structural component of the modern learning environment. In common use the concept of a 'group' can be multifaceted. Yet when viewed within the specific context of a teaching and learning strategy, the concept of 'group work' is perhaps most commonly associated with activities of small group learning (SGL). This practice involves the purposeful subdivision of any given student group into smaller subgroups (ranging in size from 2 to 20 students), with the intention of facilitating student participation and interaction with a view to attaining

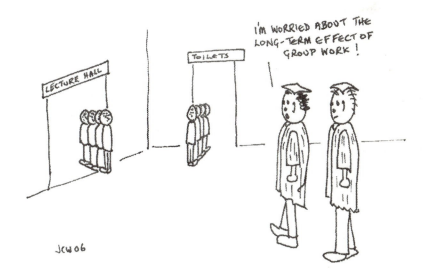

a shared learning goal. Activities associated with SGL, also referred to as cooperative learning or group discussion,[2] may include small group discussions, buzz groups, role play, scenarios, and many other such techniques (*see* Box 3.1).

As a student I can recollect experiencing many types of group work activity with varying degrees of enthusiasm. I doubt that I am alone in being able to recall an occasional feeling of reticence when asked to participate in group work activities. Sometimes this reticence was due to the delegated experimentation with group roles. For example, I remember disliking the role of scribe, as I felt that my poor spelling would be on public display. At other times the notion of being actively involved in the session just seemed too much like hard work!

In recent years I have used numerous types of SGL activities within my teaching practice with varying degrees of success. Yet despite endeavouring to ensure that the use of any teaching strategy is based on the specific learning objectives applied, I have found that I rely most heavily on two SGL activities – buzz groups and scenarios. Such a practice carries the risk of applying inappropriate teaching methods as a result of the need to feel comfortable and confident when teaching. Indeed the temptation to apply only one or two methods of group work is actively discouraged,[2] as there is a risk of students perceiving overexposure to any one teaching method. This has led me to question my knowledge of group work as a teaching strategy, and this chapter represents the results of my reflection.

BOX 3.1 Activities associated with small group learning

- Brainstorming sessions
- Buzz groups
- Cross-over groups
- Fish-bowl groups
- Free discussion
- Open-ended enquiries
- Peer tutoring
- Problem-based tutorial group
- Role play
- Self-help group
- Seminar
- Simulation/game
- Snowballing
- Step-by-step discussion
- Structured enquiries
- Syndicate
- Tutorial
- Tutorless group

(Adapted from Griffiths.[2])

Defining group work

Group work can be defined as 'co-operative work between several people.'[3] In the literature, the scope of group work is far broader than such a definition would at first indicate. Robins and Greenwood[4] have observed that the diversity associated with SGL effectively separates conservative and progressive teaching styles, and these may in turn be representative of wider organisational cultures. Conservative styles are categorised by a reliance on variants of the traditional tutorial or seminar approach. Here the method is used only to support didactic lecture-based teaching.[2,4,5] Progressive approaches to group work are more ambitious in that they may seek not only to complement the lecture, but also to challenge the premise of a lecture-based curriculum completely. Progressive approaches often seek to place the student at the centre of learning, transforming teaching from a didactic form into a participatory experience.[2] Examples include group work applied to problem-based learning[6,7] and work-based learning curricula.[8,9]

However, it is possible to identify a common denominator in all group work strategies, as there is an inherent requirement for students to learn through mutual enquiry. Scheull states:

> It is important to remember that what the student does is actually more important in determining what is learned than what the teacher does.[10]
>
> (p.429)

In practice it is possible to envisage a middle road that exists between the conservative and progressive approaches. For example, it has been suggested[1] that the interspersing of informal cooperative learning methods should occur within more traditional didactic lectures. This approach of varying teaching and learning activities within any one lesson is thought to maximise attention to any single learning method, by taking into account the student's ability to maintain concentration.[11] However, the inclusion of multiple methods introduces a risk that the tutor will use a teaching method for the sake of preventing students from becoming bored. Without a doubt any learning strategy should be applied only after careful consideration of how the methods used will match the intended learning outcomes.

Perhaps central to any discussion of group work is the need to clarify what is meant by the concept of a group. Johnson and Johnson[1] have identified numerous definitions of the concept of a group, and have reduced them to seven distinguishing characteristics (*see* Box 3.2). By amalgamating these characteristics, they propose the following definition:

> A small group is two or more individuals in face-to-face interaction, each aware of positive interdependence as they strive to achieve mutual goals, each aware of his or her membership in the group, and each aware of the others who belong to the group.[1]
>
> (p.19)

Within this definition it is possible to identify the central role of communication. Consequently, groups can be described as social structures.

The social nature of groups is further established within the definition by the recognition that group members have a 'mutual goal', but also that individuals are interdependent. This interdependence indicates that any event which affects one member of the group will to some degree affect all of them. The notion of belonging is also seen to be prominent within the definition, and emphasises a possible connection to the motivational theory proposed by Maslow.[12] An additional argument[13] is that social and cultural interactions are central to the development of individual learning. For example, it is proposed[13] that the development of language is central to lifelong learning. Through language, social interaction becomes possible, and as a consequence of this the ability to learn within social groups is strengthened.

Given the emphasis on social interaction with regard to learning, it becomes immediately apparent that teachers, when equipped with the skills necessary to manipulate group interaction, will have an advantage in helping students to learn. Griffiths[2] suggests that SGL represents one of the most highly skilled teaching activities. Not only must the tutor have a grasp of the subject that is being taught, but they must also manage a number of influences that are vital to group functioning.

An appreciation of how groups work is therefore essential for any tutor who is seeking to use SGL methods successfully. Group dynamics can be defined as the scientific study of group behaviour.[3] This includes the study of how groups are formed, and the interrelationships between individuals, groups and wider social structures.[1] Although an exploration of group dynamics is beyond the scope of this chapter, a useful first step may be to classify the types of group structures that are most commonly applied.

There are three basic types of cooperative learning, namely informal, formal and base groups.[1] These may be viewed as classification types to which a number of different learning methods (e.g. role play or scenarios) can be applied. Informal groups are set up on an ad-hoc basis during a class to help to ensure active cognitive processing of the content that is covered.[1] The use of buzz groups, in which small numbers of students (two to six) are asked to discuss a specific question or problem and give feedback, is a common method of informal cooperative learning.

Formal cooperative learning may be used to teach specific content – for example, the establishment of teams to explore a specified problem or conduct an experiment.[1] Here the focus of teaching is congruent with experiential learning theory. Instead of the teacher acting as a 'middleman' or 'conduit' between the students and the material to be covered, the teacher aims to become a facilitator, seeking to uncover the learning material *with* the students as opposed to *for* the students. This role requires the teacher to develop a non-didactic approach, and to develop a more in-depth appreciation of group dynamics. Formal types of cooperative learning require a number of pre-instructional factors to be considered. These include specifying the learning objective, the size of the groups, assigning students to groups, assigning specific roles to students, developing an assessment strategy and ensuring that an appropriate physical learning environment is available. Once planned, the task needs to be introduced to the students in a structured format. What do you expect the students to do? How will their success be measured? How are they interdependent? And what is their individual accountability? When the groups begin work, the teacher needs to monitor student behaviour with regard to interpersonal skills and academic progress. Intervention needs to be balanced and appropriate. As Johnson and Johnson[1] have stated, 'Choosing when to intervene is part of the art of teaching.'

BOX 3.2 Seven distinguishing characteristics of groups

1. *Goals.* A number of individuals join together to achieve a goal.
2. *Interdependence.* There is a collection of individuals such that an event which affects one member will to a varying degree affect all of the other members.
3. *Interpersonal interaction.* A group can be defined as a number of individuals who interact with one another.
4. *Perceptions of membership.* A group is a social unit in which individuals perceive a sense of belonging.
5. *Structured relationships.* A group is a collection of individuals who interact within the limitations imposed by established roles and norms.
6. *Mutual influence*: A group consists of individuals who influence one another.
7. *Motivation*: A group of individuals seeks to satisfy personal needs through joint association.

(Based on the categories identified by Johnson and Johnson.[1])

The final type of cooperative learning group is a 'base group.'[1] Base groups are fundamentally different from the informal and formal group structures in that they may only be applied on a long-term basis. For example, they may run for the duration of a modular study block or for an entire course. The focus of the groups is to enable students to develop long-term relationships with peers, with a threefold aim:

1 to provide ongoing support, encouragement and, where needed, assistance to one another
2 to hold each other accountable for striving to learn
3 to make sure that all members of the group are making good academic progress.

Advantages of group work

The core characteristics of groups have numerous potential advantages for learning (*see* Box 3.3), and these are reflected in the reasons why educators seek to use cooperative learning strategies. Reynolds[14] categorises the reasons for educators choosing to use SGL into three types – motivational, educational and ideological. It should be noted that educators, when considering group work activities, might use a rationale based on a mixture of these categories to justify their decision making. Furthermore, it should be noted that Reynolds does not describe these categories as an exhaustive list.

Motivational factors are simply based on the notion that students learn more when they are actively engaged and enjoying themselves.[14] Such a notion is supported by numerous other authors.[2,13,15] Furthermore, SGL offers practical advantages to the learning environment, which may positively impact on a student's motivation to engage in learning.

BOX 3.3 Potential advantages of group work

Motivational advantages
- Students can learn more as they are actively engaged.
- Activities can be fun, and this encourages learning.
- SGL uses smaller groups, so it is easier for everyone to have a say.
- SGL uses smaller groups, so others are more likely to be able to listen.
- Students can have a sense of belonging.
- Students have a shared sense of purpose.
- Students are given an opportunity to interact.
- SGL can foster a perception of peer support.

Educational advantages
- Learning in groups recognises the importance of others within the learning environment.
- Students learn more when they are actively involved in the learning process.
- Students learn through experience.
- SGL facilitates learning as a process of mutual discovery.
- Active participation in group activities can encourage a deep approach to learning.
- SGL can be used to facilitate self-directed learning.

Ideological advantages
- Many of the skills gained are transferable to work environments.
- SGL develops the following group skills:
  - communication (especially verbal skills)
  - interpersonal skills
  - negotiation
  - conflict resolution
  - problem solving
  - teamwork
  - critical thinking
  - leadership.

(Adapted from Reynolds,[14] Griffiths,[2] Maskell[3] and Reid et al.[13])

Reid and colleagues[13] have identified several such practical advantages. For example, it is easier to listen and to contribute to discussions within a group of four than it is in a class of 30 students. The advantages proposed by this argument can be closely linked to the educational theories of experiential and action learning espoused by Kolb[16] and Kember.[17] Furthermore, the active engagement of students in learning activities has been reported to have the potential to encourage students to use deep as opposed to surface approaches to learning.[18] Thus it can be demonstrated that a degree of overlap exists between the motivational and educational advantages of SGL.

Collaborative learning theory has links to the educational theories of Dewey.[1] Central to many of Dewey's educational theories is the predominant role of the learning environment. Indeed, according to Dewey an individual cannot be separated from the influence of the environment in which he exists:

> Our desires, emotions and affections are but various ways in which our doings
> are tied up with the doings of things and persons about us.[19]
>
> (p.125)

Johnson and Johnson[1] have labelled this concept 'social interdependence.' In applying SGL strategies, tutors are seeking to take advantage of the positive aspects of social interdependence, namely cooperation.

Cooperation is defined as occurring when a group of individuals is working positively towards the attainment of mutual goals,[1] and it carries numerous potential benefits for both the learner and the tutor. However, it is important to bear in mind that negative interdependence also exists, where individuals work in competition with one another. Group behaviour is therefore a complex interplay between the individual and their wider environment, including the attitudes and behaviours of others. Therefore, in order to exploit fully the advantages of SGL, the tutor must first become adept in the management of the learning environment itself. When viewed in this wider context, SGL activities become far more complex than they perhaps first appear.

If small groups are to be successful in the various activities set, then it is likely that each member of the group will need to engage actively with the desired content. Such active engagement can potentially encourage a deep approach to learning.[18] However, Griffiths[2] describes SGL as a 'highly skilled activity' in that not only must the tutor become skilled in the finer details of the content being taught, and the management of groups, but also so must the learner. This raises questions with regard to the assumptions inherent in learning theories based on the andragogical approach.

One such assumption is that students are prepared to be self-directed learners. This notion has been challenged. For example, Regan[20] has explored the concept of motivation in relation to self-directed learning (SDL), and has found the degree of student motivation to be variable, whereas Fisher and colleagues[21] describe a continuum of student readiness in relation to SDL. Given that SDL shares numerous links to experiential and action-learning theories, it becomes possible to hypothesise that students must possess good group working skills in order to realise some of the outcomes intended in the use of SGL strategies.

Paradoxically, a further advantage of the use of SGL strategies is provision of the opportunity for students to develop the skills necessary for efficient group work. This represents Reynolds' ideological category of rationale.[14] The basis here is that group structures are prominent within the workplace and wider society, and therefore the use of group work within class facilitates the development of numerous transferable skills – for example, communication skills. Consider the notion that successful groups do not simply occur, but rather they develop. Unsurprisingly, several theories of group development exist, perhaps one of the best known being that of Tuckman.[22]

Tuckman proposes a five-stage approach to group development (*see* Box 3.4), in which the behaviour of group members is influenced by the presence of specific issues. For example, the storming stage of group development is categorised by the presence of conflict within the individual members of the group, with regard to either the specific task or the influence of the group. Consequently, the management of conflict becomes the predominant focus of the group as individuals seek to confront their various differences.[1] The need to manage such a situation is said to develop the interpersonal and problem-solving skills of the individuals within the group, and this is identified as a significant advantage of SGL strategies.[9,23,24]

BOX 3.4 Tuckman's five-stage approach to group development

1. *Forming*: defining the rules and individual places within the group.
2. *Storming*: resolving conflict within the group.
3. *Norming*: reaching a consensus with regard to group structure and behaviour.
4. *Performing*: the group members become proficient in working as a unit.
5. *Adjourning*: the group separates.

Disadvantages of group work

Numerous potential disadvantages can be identified within the motivational, educational and ideological reasons for using SGL. For example, although the ideological rationale makes explicit the development of transferable skills, in application the development of group skills may be secondary to the content that is being delivered. Here there is the potential for conflict between the implicit learning outcomes attached to a lesson (representing 'added value') and the explicit learning outcomes associated with the curriculum itself (representing 'essential content'). Careful consideration is needed when selecting appropriate methods for group work, in order to avoid overloading students with potentially conflicting activities. As Eva has stated:

> Educational opportunities often succeed despite the formation of teams, not as a result.[25]
>
> (p.315)

If any group work activity places too many demands on the need to establish a working group, the likely result will be the distraction of students away from the intended content.

Connected with the motivational rationale for using SGL there are several additional disadvantages to the strategy. Of particular note is the concept of group resistance. According to Lowry,[9] a degree of group resistance is to be expected within any group work activity. Such resistance may be attributed to an apparent fixation on past issues, including the transference of past group work experience. It is important to recognise that such group resistance is not merely symptomatic of normal group development, but can indicate a more substantial problem.

Consider, for example, how a formal assessment strategy applied to SGL may also influence the degree of resistance experienced. Chin and Overton[26] have identified that formal assessment of group work has numerous potential advantages to tutors and students alike – for example, encouraging active student participation and saving the tutor time in marking. However, Elliot and Higgins[24] have indicated that problems can arise due to students perceiving the assessment process as unfair. This can happen when all of the students within a group are awarded the same grade, irrespective of their individual contribution. Unless groups are encouraged to work through the issues that are generating resistance, a demoralising and counterproductive group dynamic will probably develop.

In addition to the motivational, educational and ideological rationale,[14] two further aspects of group learning can be identified. Reynolds[14] labels these as 'frivolous' and 'getting it wrong.' The frivolous use of group work is most often exposed when the tutor decides to use group work without giving careful consideration to the suitability of the strategy – for example, the use of group work activities to cover a section of the lesson that has not been adequately prepared for by the tutor, or inclusion on the premise of giving the students something that is fun to do. Such an approach may be well intentioned, and may occasionally work well, but more often it is likely to lead to the dissatisfaction of both the student and the teacher.

The 'getting it wrong' category[14] relates to when the tutor misrepresents the group work approach. This could be through the assumption of incorrect limitations with regard to alternative learning strategies. Interestingly, Reynolds[14] cites as an example the misinterpretation that students in a lecture are passive recipients. He argues that the mental processes undertaken by students in lectures are in themselves active.

A number of authors have identified several more practical disadvantages associated with the everyday use of SGL methods. For example, a small-scale study[5] identified numerous problems associated with SGL from the perspective of both tutor and student. Within the study results, several areas of consensus between the sample groups were found to exist, namely non-attendance, dominance in participation, poor student self-confidence and reluctance to participate. Interestingly, it is suggested that the reluctance of some students to participate may place pressure on the tutor to intervene and therefore dominate the group session.[5] Tutor dominance is also identified as a potential problem in the qualitative research of Steinert,[7] which was based on students involved in problem-based learning tutorials.

Furthermore, Steinert[7] investigated what students believe makes a good group tutor. Key attributes included someone who was highly motivated and non-threatening, who could encourage group interaction and promote critical thinking and problem solving. These findings support the description of SGL as a highly skilled activity.[2] As such, it is perhaps incorrect to assume that tutor competence in the facilitation of groups can develop without the provision of appropriate support.

Summary

Group work represents a vital component in the development of student learning. This is especially the case where there is a high degree of parity between the implicit and explicit learning outcomes – for example, in teaching communication and interpersonal skills. The number and variety of available methods related to the implementation of SGL, provide a massive degree of flexibility to the tutor who is seeking to implement a high level of interaction within the learning environment. Furthermore, there is significant support for SGL approaches in educational theory.

Yet it is clear that group work as a strategy does not represent a panacea for teaching practice. In order for the strategy to prove effective, the use of group work needs to be carefully matched to the intended learning outcomes (both explicit and implicit). Therefore preparation for group work can be seen to be essential, dispelling the myth that group work strategies represent an easy option whereby the teacher can relax and let the students do the work. At the very minimum, consideration must be given to the type of group work to be used, the assessment of the group activities, and management of individual group dynamics.

- ❐ SGL promotes discussion and peer learning.
- ❐ There are numerous advantages to using group work
- ❐ Attention must be paid to the dynamics of the group.
- ❐ The main role of the tutor is one of facilitation.
- ❐ SGL is useful for any discussion where discussion and debate are required.
- ❐ Group work can be overused.

References

1 Johnson DW, Johnson FP. *Joining Together Group Theory and Group Skills.* 8th ed. London: International Student Edition, Pearson Education Ltd; 2003.
2 Griffiths S. Teaching and learning in small groups. In: Fry H, Ketteridge S, Marshall S, editors. *A Handbook for Teaching and Learning in Higher Education.* London: Taylor & Francis; 2003.
3 Maskell P. *Working in Groups: a quick guide.* Cambridge: Daniels Publishing; 1995.
4 Robins L, Greenwood J. Groups and groupwork in public administration. *Public Admin.* 2000; **78**: 957–65.
5 Boggard A, Carey SC, Dodd G *et al.* Small group teaching: perceptions and problems. *Politics.* 2005; **25**: 116–25.

6 Kropiunigg U, Pucher I, Weckenmann M. Learning in groups: teamshaping in the teaching of medical psychology. *Med Educ.* 2002; **36:** 334–6.

7 Steinert Y. Student perceptions of effective small group teaching. *Med Educ.* 2004; **38:** 286–93.

8 Rossin D, Hyland T. Groupwork-based learning within higher education: an integral ingredient for the personal and social development of students. *Mentor Tutor.* 2003; **11:** 153–62.

9 Lowry M. Working in syndicate groups towards the development of clinical protocols: a study into the professional learning of undergraduate nursing students. *Nurs Educ Today.* 1998; **18:** 470–76.

10 Shuell TJ. Cognitive conceptions of learning. *Review Educ Research.* 1986; **56:** 411–36.

11 Reece I, Walker S. *Teaching, Training and Learning: a practical guide incorporating FENTO standards.* 5th ed. Oxford: Business Education Publishers Ltd; 2003.

12 Maslow AH. *Motivation and Personality.* London: Harper & Rowe; 1954.

13 Reid J, Forrestal P, Cook J. *Small Group Learning in the Classroom.* Scarborough, WA: Chalkface Press; 1989.

14 Reynolds M. *Groupwork in Education and Training: ideas in practice.* London: Kogan Page; 1994.

15 Tiberius R. *Small Group Teaching: a trouble-shooting guide.* London: Kogan Page; 1999.

16 Kolb DA. *Experiential Learning: experience as the source of learning and development.* Englewood Cliffs, NJ: Prentice Hall; 1984.

17 Kember D. *Action Learning and Action Research: improving the quality of teaching and learning.* London: Kogan Page; 2000.

18 Gibbs G. *Improving the Quality of Student Learning.* Bristol: Technical and Educational Services; 1992.

19 Dewey J. *Democracy and Education;* www.netLibrary.com (accessed 7 June 2004).

20 Regan JA. Motivating students towards self-directed learning. *Nurs Educ Today.* 2003; **23:** 593–9.

21 Fisher M, King J, Tague G. Development of a self-directed learning readiness scale for nursing education. *Nurs Educ Today.* 2001; **21:** 516–25.

22 Tuckman BW. Developmental sequence in small groups. *Psychol Bull.* 1965; **63:** 384–99; reprinted online at http://dennislearningcenter.osu.edu/references/ GROUP%20DEV%20ARTICLE.doc (accessed 22 January 2006).

23 Huxham M, Land R. Assigning students to group work projects. Can we do better than random? *Innovations Educ Train Int.* 2000; **37:** 17–22.

24 Elliot N, Higgins A. Self and peer assessment: does it make a difference to student group work? *Nurs Educ Pract.* 2005; **5:** 40–48.

25 Eva KW. Teamwork during education: the whole is not always greater than the sum of the parts. *Med Educ.* 2002; **36:** 314–16.

26 Chin P, Overton T. *Assessing Group Work: advice and examples.* The Higher Education Academy Physical Sciences Centre, Primer 6, Version 2, issued March 2005; www. physsci.heacademy.ac.uk/publications/primer/group6.pdf

CHAPTER 4

Problem-based learning

Jan Gidman and Jean Mannix

This chapter will be written from the perspective of two lecturers within a School of Health and Social Care. Jan has been using problem-based learning with students for many years, mainly within pre-registration nursing programmes, whereas Jean has only recently entered teaching and become involved with problem-based learning, mainly with post-registration students. At their first meeting to discuss this chapter, they had an interesting debate about their different experiences of the nature of students and the use of problem-based learning.

Jean first encountered problem-based learning when she was a practice mentor for health-visiting students, although she did not realise at the time that she was using any specific teaching and learning strategy. This involved setting the scene of a client in health visiting and following through a client journey, using triggers and issues raised to stimulate learning in relation to real-life situations. As a novice lecturer,

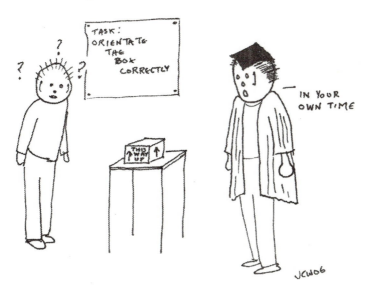

Jean used case studies and scenarios on a regular basis, because she was familiar and comfortable with this approach and her own teaching style is one of facilitation rather than 'chalk and talk.'

Jan had a very different introduction to problem-based learning when she started her first post in higher education and became involved in an undergraduate degree programme for nurses, using an approach to problem-based learning to underpin the adult branch of the curriculum. This approach will be explained in the following section, which considers definitions of problem-based learning. Again this fitted Jan's own teaching and learning style, which was to be student-centred and practice-orientated.

As Jean explored the theoretical basis of problem-based learning within her Postgraduate Diploma in Education programme, she gained confidence and used this approach increasingly as a teaching and learning strategy with students on the Specialist Practitioner Qualification (SPQ) programme and with practice-based mentors. An example of a setting where this was used very effectively was a two-day 'safeguarding children' workshop within the SPQ programme. One of the major drivers for this was the Government agenda with regard to inter-professional learning – in this case practice nurses, district nurses, learning disability nurses, school nurses and health visitors. The workshop was facilitated by a health visitor (Jean), a mental health lecturer and a social worker. Jean's knowledge of problem-based learning identified it as the most appropriate strategy for promoting inter-professional learning. The composition and experience of the student group meant that problem-based learning facilitated the sharing of knowledge and experience, and it also encouraged individuals to explore attitudes and break down professional barriers.

CASE STUDY 4.1

Jean's current role also involves the preparation and support of mentors in the community. These mentors are experienced practitioners who promote learning and assess students on the SPQ programme. Jean developed scenarios in relation to failing students in practice, which had been highlighted as an issue of concern for mentors. She asked a colleague to review these in terms of whether they would promote discussion and debate between mentors (experienced and novice mentors from a range of pathways). This colleague telephoned the next day and said that she had discussed the scenarios and debated the range of options and perspectives all evening, and was very excited about using them with mentors. When Jean actually used the scenarios, she decided to include cues and triggers to guide the students, to ensure that they understood the university guidance and process to fail students. At the time, this was considered to be a successful session and was well evaluated by participants. However, experience of using the same scenario again with a different mentor group, but this time without the cues, led to a much richer debate, which was not constrained by predetermined outcomes.

Jan's experience of using problem-based learning has been mainly with pre-registration nursing students, initially with small groups of students and later using an adaptation of problem-based learning, namely scenario-generated learning, with large groups of students. These two approaches will be discussed in the following section, which explores definitions and some of the applications of problem-based learning.

When Jan and Jean discussed the writing of this chapter, it led to a significant debate about the use of problem-based learning in pre-registration programmes, which are inherently outcome-driven due to professional standards and competencies.

One of the challenges that Jan had faced when she moved to her current post was the need to implement the applied sciences modules within a pre-registration nursing programme using a problem-based learning approach. This involved integrating biology, sociology and psychology, which had previously been delivered as separate entities. Although these were applied to real-life scenarios, it was difficult to implement true problem-based learning due to the large size of the student groups and the time and resource constraints. The resource implications in terms of lecturers, classrooms, information technology and library access will be discussed later in the chapter in relation to the potential disadvantages of problem-based learning.

As Jan and Jean discussed their experiences of using problem-based learning, it became evident that not only did the term include a range of approaches, but also there was wide variation in its application according to student group, in this case between pre-registration nursing students and post-registration experienced practitioners and mentors.

Defining problem-based learning

Problem-based learning was originally developed within medical education,[1] and is currently incorporated in many undergraduate medical curricula, including those in the UK.[2] Problem-based learning was adopted in nurse education in Australia, where it was initially used to underpin the entire curriculum.[3] More recently, problem-based learning has been widely adopted within health education in the UK, although here it is used as a learning and teaching strategy rather than as a curriculum approach.[4,5] Many universities in Australia have also moved away from delivering the entire curriculum in this way, due to the major time and resource implications.

Barrows and Tamblyn[1] were two of the principal creators of the problem-based learning approach that was introduced at MacMaster University, and they offer the following definition:

> problem-based learning is the learning that results from the process of working toward the understanding or resolution of a problem. The problem is encountered first in the learning process![1]

(p.1)

Barrows and Tamblyn suggest that problem-based learning is not simply the presentation of problems as a focus for learning, but rather it involves a very specific approach to education, which is supported by tools designed to support the teaching–learning process. Indeed, Barrows and Tamblyn claim that:

> problem-based, student-centred learning is the most efficient method of simul-taneously developing knowledge, reasoning skills and study skills.[1]
>
> (p.xiii)

Although the method was designed for use in medical education, Barrows and Tamblyn[1] argue that problem-based learning is relevant and appropriate to other healthcare professionals, because it will enable them to apply their knowledge and enhance their practice. Jean and Jan's experience of utilising problem-based learning reflects these claims. Students were self-directed and took responsibility for their scenario, and the application of theory to practice was indeed enhanced. Problem-based learning can be undertaken using a seven-step approach (*see* Box 4.1).[6,7] A fundamental requirement when planning the scenario is that it addresses the learning outcomes that need to be achieved. A variety of triggers can be utilised to enhance or promote the problem-based learning process, including photographs, video clips, poetry, music and literature. These would form a package of problem-based triggers to generate interest and motivation and to challenge students' creativity.[6,7] Currency of the specialist area is vital, and the inclusion of practitioners and mentors to develop the scenarios and triggers enhances the experience for students by bringing real-world practice into the classroom.

BOX 4.1 Seven-step approach to problem-based learning

1. Students are allocated to small, mixed groups of six to eight, according to their professional and educational experience.
2. A scenario is read to the students by the lecturer, and they are given an individual copy of the scenario.
3. Students are asked whether they understand the vocabulary and are given the opportunity to clarify any issues.
4. A student is appointed by the team to act as a scribe, to record the discussions and issues raised.
5. A chair is appointed, who may also be the scribe, to steer the group and to encourage discussion, exploration and clarification if needed.
6. Students identify issues and implement an action plan. This may involve further individual or group work.
7. Students then share and integrate with the group any knowledge gained, and evaluate this knowledge in the context of the scenario.

(Adapted from David and Patel[6] and Wilkie and Burns.[7])

The literature describes differences in the application of problem-based learning. At one extreme it is advocated as the main focus of the curriculum and is the whole philosophy of learning,[1] and at the other end of the continuum it is one of a range of learning and teaching strategies.

The problem-based learning approach that Jan first encountered was the hypothetico-deductive approach, as developed at the MacArthur Institute of Higher Education, New South Wales, Australia.[4] This approach uses the framework of a simulated situation and is designed to develop students' analytical skills by a process of logical deduction. It relies on students developing hypotheses from the presented problem scenario and then assessing the validity of each hypothesis against the given facts. If sufficient facts are not available to test the hypotheses, students need to obtain whatever further information is necessary to enable them to determine which hypothesis is most appropriate.

Students were initially presented with scenarios that required their intervention as practitioners. They were required to search the literature to find relevant theories and then to use critical thinking and decision-making skills to identify best practice in each particular case. Six problem studies were developed to meet specific module learning outcomes and to reflect the central concepts of the curriculum. Scenarios were based on real-life situations, which have been shown to stimulate more interest among students.[7]

Knowles[8] contends that adult learners prefer immediacy of application to ensure that learning is relevant. This has implications for curriculum development, which should ensure that the sequencing of learning facilitates this, in order to maximise the integration of theory and practice. Problem-based learning is a strategy which, in both Jan's and Jean's experience, can contribute effectively to this.

The advantages of problem-based learning

Problem-based learning as a teaching strategy has its underpinning historical influences within medical education.[5,7,9] Ryan[10] advises that problem-based learning can provide high-quality outcomes for learning, but recommends that in order to achieve this, the learning should be realistic and adequate time and resources should be available for students to undertake self-directed learning. It is well documented in the medical literature that the philosophy of problem-based learning facilitates inter-professional learning, while relating theory to practice to produce 'knowledgeable doers.'[11,12] Bearing this in mind, it seemed appropriate to use problem-based learning as a strategy for specialist practice students. As the fundamental philosophy of problem-based learning is andragogy, this supported its relevance as a learning and teaching strategy for experienced practitioners undertaking post-registration study.[5,7]

There are constant demands from the Department of Health, professional bodies and Government policies in terms of the changing roles of health and social care practitioners. In order to meet the demands of an ever-changing profession, health and social care education needs to meet these challenges and confront professional boundaries. Working together is now a fundamental requirement within health and social care, and it is therefore logical to facilitate inter-professional learning within education programmes. Problem-based learning has a theme of inter-professional learning and collaboration. This then would set the scene for the student's progression into real-world practice.[13]

Problem-based learning has the potential to provide the necessary learning climate for health education.[5,7,14] The strategy emphasises problem solving in real-world practice, because the process encourages learners to explore and find solutions within a safe environment.[15] This should help to prepare practitioners to work within team dynamics, playing to their own and other team members' strengths, improving teamwork and consequently promoting their capacity to function in teams. This will ensure a good foundation to promote health and social care professionals who are fit for practice and purpose in the ever-changing National Health Service.[16]

Health education was traditionally driven by an outcome-led curriculum, which is divided by subject and discipline.[13] However, problem-based learning is an holistic teaching strategy that views clients as individuals, with individual needs and problems. By exploring triggers within a problem-based learning approach, the process may enhance critical thinking skills and decision making.[13] This subject integration and holism is considered to be a particular strength of problem-based learning within the education of healthcare professionals.

With a shift in the demands of healthcare, educators need to re-evaluate existing teaching and learning strategies[17] in order to ensure that health education maintains its momentum and enables practitioners to meet future as well as current demands. Problem-based learning explores approaches that promote the student's growth and development, and is therefore deemed to be a platform for lifelong learning.[14]

When problem-based learning was utilised in the 'safeguarding children' workshop, the learning became more relevant and challenging both for students and for lecturers.[15] This increased student and lecturer motivation and helped to bridge the theory–practice gap for students.[5] The SPQ students on the workshop confirmed this within their evaluations, stating that:

> Case studies were thought provoking, brought the subject to life.

> Helpful to share ideas, I was pleased the case studies were relevant to each discipline, allowing the opportunity to link theory to practice.

These quotes also confirm the findings of the descriptive study by Carey and Whittaker,[14] in which 79% of students said that they valued the opportunity to explore real practice, which suggested that problem-based learning brought the theoretical perspectives to life.

Within the SPQ programme, the 'safeguarding children' workshop included students from all pathways. Problem-based learning was utilised as a strategy to promote discussion and for students to share their experience and knowledge. The scenarios were written jointly with a social worker and lecturer who both had experience of practice issues. The students were asked to form multi-disciplinary groups, each consisting of eight students, to discuss the main issues of the scenario and compile a multi-agency action plan, as suggested within the problem-based learning strategy, to ensure varied knowledge and skills. The key themes that emerged both during the session and in the evaluations were shared learning and collaborative working practices. These are particularly relevant to community nursing. Examples from students' evaluations are given below:

> I enjoyed working collaboratively with other students. I learnt a great deal from the others.

> Thought I knew it all about child protection. In fact I learnt a lot about others' (nurses and social workers) roles, responsibilities and referral pathways.

The facilitation of problem-based learning is a balancing process – too much or too little intervention can suppress the process of problem-based learning.[18] Within the workshop this balancing process proved difficult, as it is possible to become over-involved, which can detract from the students' learning experience. It is necessary to ensure that students are responsible for their own learning, to further enhance their growth, development and confidence.[13]

The student-centred approach, rather than a traditional teacher-centred strategy, was fundamental to the workshop to encourage deeper learning.[19] Knowles[8] purports that supporting learners in the andragogical process can encourage students to believe in their own ability, which will give them confidence to learn more successfully.[20]

Students felt that the problem-based learning experience provided realism and safety within the case studies, which would give them confidence in practice. Carey and Whittaker[14] support this view, reporting that the development of self-directed learning skills promoted within problem-based learning is beneficial to community nurses. These skills prepare students for real-world practice, which can be isolating and unpredictable in the community environment, requiring critical thinking and autonomous practice.[21] This is highlighted by the following quote from the 'safeguarding children' workshop evaluation:

> It was very useful having social and health perspective throughout the day, setting the scene for future practice.

The rationale for exploring problem-based learning within the context of specialist practice was that specialist practitioner students are generally mature, experienced learners with a diverse range of knowledge and experiences. It would seem shrewd to embrace the wealth of rich knowledge that some students possess, to share with other practitioners, thereby promoting inter-professional learning. The study by Carey and Whittaker[14] recognised that problem-based learning encouraged students to share and reflect on their experiences of clinical practice. This provides the opportunity for students to deconstruct ideas through the process of problem-based learning and reflection, generating innovative theories which can then be implemented within practice placements.

The disadvantages of problem-based learning

The literature explores a number of potential disadvantages or challenges associated with the use of problem-based learning as a learning and teaching strategy. These will now be explored in relation to health and social care education.

Assessment of learning is a major issue in health and social care education, and has two main aims, namely the personal development of the student and the professional selection of students who meet the required competencies. It is suggested that the outcome requirements of professional qualification currently take precedence over the individual development of the student.[22] In line with the principles of andragogy, problem-based learning approaches would involve each student being assessed against his or her own goals, rather than applying a standard assessment format to the whole group.[1] This could be a major constraint on the use of the method to assess professional outcomes, particularly with large cohorts of students.

The use of problem-based learning within any curriculum has major implications for the role of lecturers. This andragogical approach requires that lecturers are student-centred and promote learning, rather than delivering subject matter, and it has been argued that adult education has not reached its full potential because many lecturers are unfamiliar with the approach.[8]

In Jan's experience of using problem-based learning with pre-registration nursing students, the latter felt that they had learned most from sessions, and had found them most valuable, when she had been least directive and had encouraged them to explore the issues that they themselves had identified as relevant. This is consistent with Jean's experience with regard to deciding not to use cues for students. However, one experience in particular illustrates the tensions between an outcome-driven curriculum and a problem-based learning approach (*see* Case study 4.2).

CASE STUDY 4.2

Using the hypothetico-deductive method described previously, Jan introduced a group of students to a scenario relating to breast cancer. The scenario described the experience of a woman who, having discovered a breast lump, was admitted for surgery following a fine-needle aspiration. The students identified, and focused on, the initial diagnosis and its effect on the woman and her family, whereas the lecturers who were developing the scenario, and indeed the curriculum outcomes, focused on surgical intervention! This caused great concern initially, but the team very quickly decided to let the group pursue their issues, and to find an alternative way of addressing the other outcomes. This led to unexpected but valid responses from the students, and to learning and a change in perspective for the lecturers involved – not just in terms of the priorities in caring for a woman with breast cancer, but also in terms of the value of problem-based learning. Reflecting on the experience, I am also aware that these problem-based learning sessions shifted the balance of power from lecturers to students, and that the learning was truly student-centred.

As lecturers using this approach, we need to 'expect the unexpected', encourage this, and value the learning that we also gain during the process. Andrews and Jones[4] argue that it is difficult for lecturers to achieve an effective balance between non-participation and active facilitation. It is sometimes necessary for the facilitator to interject or 'call time out', but if interruptions are too frequent there is a danger that the power base, and responsibility for learning, will shift back from the students to the lecturer.

A common misconception with regard to student-centred approaches to education is that it means 'leaving students to it'! On the contrary, these approaches require increased time and commitment from lecturers, and considerable skill to facilitate students' ability to be self-directed in their learning.[23] Little[24] has described an action research project that identifies some of the important factors in the implementation of problem-based learning. These include lecturers having an understanding of (and commitment to) the philosophy of the approach, a realistic acceptance of the role change, the ability to model critical thinking and problem-solving skills, and an acceptance that students need time to change their expectations of the learning process.

The literature advises that preparation and support of lecturers who facilitate problem-based learning represent a vital issue that needs to be addressed if the strategy is to be used effectively.[1,4,25] Barrows and Tamblyn[1] cite an old oriental philosophy to explain the lecturer's role in facilitating problem-based learning: 'give me a fish and I eat for a day; teach me to fish and I eat for a lifetime.' Although this is consistent with the requirement for health and social care practitioners to become lifelong learners, it is suggested that many lecturers find it difficult and stressful to relinquish the power inherent in traditional roles.[18]

Organisational issues are major constraints associated with problem-based learning. Extensive educational resources are required, and the curriculum needs to be structured in such a way as to allow the student to use these resources as he or she feels appropriate, and to set the pace of the learning. Problem-based learning needs close cooperation between members of all the disciplines involved, and requires adequate classroom space and small group sizes. This has cost and resource implications, and it is argued that this limits its successful implementation within higher education institutions.[5]

Another potential disadvantage of problem-based learning that has been identified in the literature is that it may not provide the same level of knowledge as traditional strategies.[26] A review of evaluative studies by Vernon and Blake[27] reported that medical students valued problem-based learning as a learning strategy, and were found to have improved clinical skills and self-directed abilities, but reduced factual knowledge in basic science, compared with traditional students.

This may lead us to ask which we value most – the process or the product of learning. As with any learning and teaching strategy, it is important to understand how the strategy will influence the learning that is to take place. Jean feels that problem-based learning is an ideal strategy for post-registration students, as many practitioners have the problem-solving and reflective skills, coupled with real-world practice, when they embark on a programme of study. The ability to engage in critical thinking and higher levels of judgement is key to the success of problem-based learning. This is slightly different within pre-registration education programmes, where students do not have the experience of Jean's SPQ students. However, an increasing number of mature students with a wealth of both life and practical experience are now entering health and social care programmes. It is vital that pre-registration programmes enable students to develop the skills that will promote lifelong learning, if they are to be effective in their professional roles. This means that curricula must promote the process of learning, rather than prioritising learning outcomes and professional competencies.

An evaluative study of nursing students by Andrews and Jones[4] also highlights potential difficulties in relation to problem-based learning. It was reported that although students assimilated large volumes of information, this was often not in sufficient depth to meet course requirements. Crucial literature was sometimes not accessed, and at times discussion remained at a superficial level. Another pertinent issue raised by Andrews and Jones[4] is that there is little evidence to support the assumption that problem-solving strategies that are used in an education setting are transferred to practice settings. They also note that in problem-based learning the students are presented with the problem, whereas in real-life settings, health and social care professionals need first to identify the problem. These authors contend that the crucial stage of problem identification is often omitted in health and social care education, and they suggest that strategies to enhance the recognition and prioritisation of problems in practice would strengthen the process.

Conclusion/summary

While writing this chapter, both authors reflected on the value and challenges of problem-based learning as a learning and teaching strategy, and it became apparent that they had very different experiences of the approach.

Jean found that problem-based learning encouraged students and mentors to have fun learning, made the process meaningful to practice and helped to bridge the theory–practice gap. It also enabled learners to gain experience, acquire transferable skills and develop the ability to reflect in action. The problem-based learning approach emphasised to Jean that the level and experience of the learners had a major impact on the success of the strategy. Bechtel and colleagues[15] have commented that learning is a 'beautiful exploration', which becomes of superlative quality when students are given a meaningful challenge that is relevant to clinical practice. This was exactly the response that Jean found with the learners (who were all experienced practitioners) when she was facilitating problem-based learning. Cooke and Mayle[28] concur that if learning is active, fun, purposeful and meaningful, students will undertake deep learning. Actively participating in a learning process promotes the students' integration and synthesis of knowledge, thus promoting problem solving and critical thinking.[28] This is a fundamental component of problem-based learning, as it is a student-centred strategy. However, students can find it a daunting prospect when they have little experience of their chosen pathway.

When using problem-based learning with pre-registration students, Jan encountered many of the challenges that have been reported in the literature. Large cohorts of students had to be divided into a number of small groups, which had major implications for resources in terms of lecturers, classrooms, library access and computer facilities. However, despite these challenges, the students evaluated the approach very positively, reporting that it encouraged them to relate theory to practice.

Problem-based learning is student-centred and based on cognitive learning psychology.[5,25] The assumption therefore is that students are active learners who construct knowledge in their own individual way. Problem-based learning is seen as an approach to learning that results from the process of working towards understanding or resolving a problem. Therefore, by placing learners at the heart of their learning experience, this approach is perceived to support professional practice, as it requires implementation as well as theoretical knowledge.

In conclusion, problem-based learning may be an ideal teaching strategy for specialist practice students. In general, students who are undertaking specialist practice qualification are experienced practitioners who have a wealth of rich knowledge to share with their peers. Due to the interdisciplinary nature of the specialist practitioner course, the students often find that they are working with prospective colleagues. Problem-based learning can increase the students' confidence in many areas of specialist practice – for example, inter-professional working, collaboration, teamwork and enhanced interpersonal skills – due to the dynamics of group work, which is the foundation of this teaching and learning strategy. Other areas that are enhanced by problem-based learning are the higher-level skills of critical thinking and decision making which are essential for practitioners in an ever changing and dynamic healthcare arena.

However, we would caution against the widespread adoption of problem-based learning within pre-registration programmes. Jan and Jean's experience has demonstrated the effectiveness of this learning strategy in integrating theory and practice and developing critical thinking and problem-solving skills in students. To facilitate this, it is important to address the major resource implications and to prepare both students and lecturers for the approach. As Milligan[23] has pointed out, problem-based learning is not a panacea, and it would be a mistake to limit the curricula and to rely on one strategy to take health and social care forward.

- ❏ Problem-based learning is a valuable strategy for promoting learning in health and social care programmes.
- ❏ Problem-based learning is process-driven rather than outcome-driven. It promotes critical thinking, reflection and problem-solving skills.
- ❏ Problem-based learning is student-centred and requires a change of role for some lecturers – to become facilitators rather than teachers.
- ❏ In order to be effective, problem-based learning requires extensive preparation of both students and facilitators.
- ❏ Problem-based learning is not an easy option – it is expensive in terms of staff, time and resources.

References

1 Barrows HS, Tamblyn RM. *Problem-Based Learning: an approach to medical education.* New York: Springer; 1980.
2 Maudsley G. Roles and responsibilities of the problem-based learning tutor in the undergraduate medical curriculum. *BMJ.* 1999; **318:** 657–61.
3 Creedy D, Horsfall J, Hand B. Problem-based learning in nurse education: an Australian view. *J Adv Nurs.* 1992; **17:** 727–33.
4 Andrews M, Jones PR. Problem-based learning in an undergraduate nursing programme: a case study. *J Adv Nurs.* 1996; **23:** 357–65.
5 Frost M. An analysis of the scope and value of problem-based learning in the education of healthcare professionals. *J Adv Nurs.* 1996; **24:** 1047–53.
6 David TJ, Patel L. Adult learning theory, problem-based learning and paediatrics. *Arch Dis Child.* 1995; **73:** 357–63.
7 Wilkie K, Burns I. *Problem-Based Learning: a handbook for nurses.* London: Palgrave; 2003.
8 Knowles M. *The Adult Learner: a neglected species.* 4th ed. Houston, TX: Gulf Publishing Co.; 1990.
9 Barrow EJ, Lyte G, Butterworth T. An evaluation of problem-based learning in a nursing theory and practice module. *Nurs Educ Pract.* 2002; **2:** 55–62.
10 Ryan G. Ensuring that students develop an adequate, well-structured knowledge base. In: Boud D, Feletti G, editors. *The Challenge of Problem-Based Learning.* 2nd ed. London: Kogan Page; 1997.
11 Department of Health. *Making a Difference: strengthening the nursing, midwifery and health visiting contribution to health and health care.* London: The Stationery Office; 1999.
12 Maudsley G, Strivens J. Promoting professional knowledge, experiential learning and critical thinking for medical students. *Med Educ.* 2000; **34:** 535–44.
13 Biley FC, Smith KL. Exploring the potential of problem-based learning in nurse education. *Nurs Educ Today.* 1998; **18:** 353–61.
14 Carey L, Whittaker KA. Experiences of problem-based learning: issues for community specialist practitioners. *Nurs Educ Today.* 2002; **22:** 661–7.

15 Bechtel GA, Davidhizar R, Bradshaw M. Problem-based learning in a competency-based world. *Nurs Educ Today*. 1999; **19**: 182–7.

16 Nursing and Midwifery Council. *Requirements for Pre-Registration Nurse Programmes*. London: Nursing and Midwifery Council; 2002.

17 Nelson L, Sadler L, Surtees G. Bringing problem-based learning to life using virtual reality. *Nurs Educ Pract*. 2005; **5**: 103–8.

18 Haith-Cooper M. Problem-based learning within health professional education. What is the role of the lecturer? A review of the literature. *Nurs Educ Today*. 2000; **20**: 267–72.

19 Biggs J. *Teaching for Quality Learning at University*. Buckingham: Open University Press; 2003.

20 Reece I, Walker S. *Teaching, Training and Learning: a practical guide incorporating FENTO standards*. 5th ed. Sunderland: Business Education Publishers; 2003.

21 Nursing and Midwifery Council. *Standards of Proficiency for Specialist Community Public Health Nurses*. London: Nursing and Midwifery Council; 2004.

22 Purdy M. The problem of self-assessment in nurse education. *Nurs Educ Today*. 1997; **17**: 135–9.

23 Milligan F. Beyond the rhetoric of problem-based learning: emancipatory limits and links with andragogy. *Nurs Educ Today*. 1999; **19**: 548–55.

24 Little S. Preparing tertiary teachers for problem-based learning. In: Boud D, Feletti G, editors. *The Challenge of Problem-Based Learning*. 2nd ed. London: Kogan; 1997.

25 Creedy D, Hand B. The implementation of problem-based learning: changing pedagogy in nurse education. *J Adv Nurs*. 1994; **20**: 696–702.

26 Albanese MA, Mitchell S. Problem-based learning: a review of literature on its outcomes and implementation issues. *Acad Med*. 1993; **68**: 52–81.

27 Vernon DT, Blake RL. Does problem-based learning work? A meta-analysis of evaluative research. *Acad Med*. 1993; **68**: 550–63.

28 Cooke M, Mayle K. Students' evaluation of problem-based learning. *Nurs Educ Today*. 2002; **22**: 330–39.

CHAPTER 5

Case study: a stilted tool or a useful learning and teaching strategy?

Sue Padmore

Reflection

The concept of case study may conjure up different things to different people. In its simplest format a case study may be very limited in content and offer a very directive approach to the student. However, more intricate case studies can be overlaid with influences of themes from the practice area, enabling further exploration and reflection on previous and future practice. In my experience, working in the sexual health field and now within higher education, case studies have proved a useful tool for stimulating discussion and debate on sensitive issues. I have found that using case studies allowed objectivity, so that students felt more able to share their beliefs,

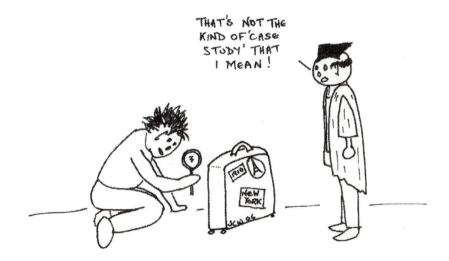

attitudes and experiences from a professional stance (although some chose to use personal examples).

I chose case study as a tool for carrying out training with registered midwives who had been informed, due to changes in the political and healthcare arenas, that they would now be expected to carry out human immunodeficiency virus (HIV) pre-test discussion as part of their role. This was my first experience of working with this group of professionals. I was also aware that they might be reluctant participants, as their presence had been decreed by managers, as part of designated, mandatory training. I knew from discussions with other colleagues that some of them had reservations about encompassing HIV pre-test discussion as part of their work role, for various reasons. I was therefore acutely aware of the need for gentle and sensitive exploration of feelings during the training sessions. That said, I needed to test their attitudinal standpoints in order to try to capture an image of how they would impart and translate the information to their clients/patients.

I decided to create four case studies based on real-life situations that I, or other health professionals working in sexual health, had encountered. The training took place over a six-month period, and therefore each group was inherently different with regard to their individual dynamics. Thus the resulting discussions and debates arising from the case studies were specific to each group. It became very clear to me early on in the programme where the concerns lay. Many midwives felt that their knowledge of HIV and AIDS was insufficient for them to support clients/patients who were receiving an HIV-positive diagnosis. They were also unsure about the process of giving positive results, as this had yet to be agreed. The sessions were evaluated positively, which suggested that the midwives valued the support that was given during the sessions and also the ongoing support that was offered on a continuing basis for their future practice needs.

CASE STUDY EXAMPLE

You have been asked by the GP to see a 24-year-old woman, Mary, for booking. Mary has a little boy from a previous relationship and is now expecting her second child. Her current partner is an intravenous drug user.

What do you think?

What do you feel?

What issues would you consider when booking this woman?

Defining case study

There are a myriad teaching and learning strategies available for use within professional education. It is suggested that taking an andragogical approach to education is essential for adult learners, with experiential learning as one of the components of andragogy.[1] Experiential learning and small group teaching are inextricably linked.[2] Group work acts as a vehicle for experiential learning to take place, with case studies, games or role play being used to enhance the learning.[1] Often students have considerable work and life experience which can be utilised to enhance effective learning within groups.

In their research, Reece and Walker[3] found that group work was actually cited as the number one teaching strategy that students preferred. It is suggested that group size and the needs, ability and motivation of students are important evidence of justification for the choice of teaching strategy.[3] I would agree that this needs careful consideration if effective learning is to take place. Group work in the form of case study allows exploration of and reflection on issues from previous practice. It also allows exploration of thoughts and feelings with regard to future practice.

Students are at the centre of learning. They view the world from their own perspective and consequently will control their own learning despite what the teacher expects them to learn from their teaching.[4] Case study can facilitate learning as it encourages interaction both with the characters in the scenario and with group members. Education is about conceptual change, and there are four important criteria that enable this to occur:[4]

■ clarity of the objectives
■ students wanting to learn (or if not, the teacher being able to motivate them)
■ students being 'on task'
■ good dialogue with peers and teachers.

All of these criteria can be applied through the use of case study.

There is a long and respectable history of the case study method of teaching within various professions and disciplines.[5] Case studies provoke discussion and provide a beneficial learning experience and exploration of clinical issues and experience. The use of case study is an effective mechanism for bringing 'real-life' experience into the classroom.[6] It is further suggested that case studies allow students to integrate their knowledge of biological, behavioural and nursing sciences.[2,7]

The advantages of case study

Quinn[2] suggests that small group work can expand the student's universe of awareness as a result of the process of events that go on within the group. This certainly echoes my own experience of people learning from each other and their individual experiences, as well as from the case studies. It is believed that the higher-level, cognitive and affective domains are more applicable to small group work.[3] This was indeed evident in the way in which students worked. It is further suggested that small group work can help students to develop the interactive and collaborative skills necessary for employment and research.[2] In my experience, the use of case studies within small group work allowed students to develop their interactive, assertive, verbal and cognitive skills.

Galileo (cited by Neary) believed that:

> You can't teach a man anything, you can only help him find it within himself.[1]

(p.93)

Learning occurs when a person makes sense of what he encounters or experiences in interacting with himself, others and the environment.[1] Learners are intrinsically different and have different preferred learning styles, whereas teaching is a purposeful activity with the aims of promoting learning and causing learning to happen.[3] As teachers we need to be aware of the diversity of our students both as individuals and within groups – group dynamics can alter an individual's responses. There are various identified learning styles cited within the literature. Honey and Mumford[3] identified four main learning styles – activists, reflectors, theorists and pragmatists. Thus students may learn in very different ways and therefore a variety of teaching tools and strategies will need to be used. This will allow them to learn and become involved in activities, and will also promote enthusiasm and increase motivation. It is impossible to choose the correct teaching strategy to suit every learning style, so it is important to use a variety of teaching strategies throughout a module or curriculum, so that every student has the same learning opportunities and their motivation and interest are maintained. The case study thus becomes another tool that teachers can use in this quest.

Kolb's learning cycle has been influential within healthcare education planning.[2] If we apply it to case study activity, the 'concrete experience' could be viewed as a second-hand experience (via the case study), the 'structured activity' could be developed through observations and reflections, the formation of 'abstract concepts and generalisations' could be developed through feedback to groups on findings, and finally the 'testing implications of concepts in new situations' could be construed as how the group respond.

When I use case study I observe the students engaging with the second-hand experience. The students recall their observations and reflections, with occasional guidance from myself. Formation of abstract concepts and generalisations takes place during the feedback to the large group, reporting findings and solutions to the issues raised within the case studies. Testing of the implications of concepts in new situations occurs as the response of students to the whole exercise. I found that their response was positive. They appeared to be motivated and enjoyed the experience of working with case study in pursuit of their learning.

This type of learning could be described as cooperative or collaborative learning.[8] Cooperative learning is the learning of new material that is initially presented by the teacher, with the group then taking responsibility for organisation of their own learning. The group members encourage one another. An extension of cooperative learning is collaborative learning, which builds on cooperative learning by creating an environment in which students work together to accomplish a task (or tasks) that they may not be able to accomplish individually.[8] There are numerous studies which show that the student-centred approach increases learning, motivation to learn and performance.[9] Tudor suggests that:

> The creativity inherent in student-centred activities adds an element of surprise to each class.[9]

I feel that due to changing group dynamics this is inevitable and is to be welcomed as a challenge by the teacher.

The literature supports the requirement for learning to be active – not only through intellectual activity, but also in physical movement. Active learning through physical movement encourages the utilisation of kinaesthetic intelligence, which can help to increase the effectiveness of memory and therefore aid reflection on practice.[10] The use of a case study requires the students to move into groups and handle the written material. It is further reported that active learning removes the passive role and provides an environment in which skills can be developed.[10] Students retain information for longer and are able to store and recall it more easily. Problem-solving abilities, initiative and students' self-esteem can all be enhanced through student-centred activities.[10] The problem-solving aspects of a case study require the student to reflect on their previous experience.

Reflection is defined as follows:

> a process of internally examining and exploring an issue of concern triggered by an experience, which creates and clarifies meaning in terms of self and results in a changed conceptual perspective.[11]

It is suggested that reflection on activity helps professionals to understand the complex and highly contextual situations that they may encounter in practice.[1] It is also thought that reflective practice allows deeper analysis to occur and encourages internalisation, which is an effective mode of learning.[1]

The contextual variability of human interaction can be examined through reflection, as this often differs from the textbook descriptions.[12] In higher education, reflection is encouraged. However, we need to be aware that this is a learned skill and one that takes time to practise. Reflection gives us insight into events and activities that we encounter throughout our working lives. It also allows a deeper level of learning.

A distinction has been made between deep and surface levels of processing.[11] Students who focus attention on specific facts or pieces of information which are rote learned in order to pass an examination or assignment have been described as having a 'surface approach' to learning. Students who take a more constructive, analytical view, such as that offered through the use of case study, have been described as having a 'deep approach' to learning.[11] It has been found that students who feel anxious or threatened are more likely to take a surface approach to learning.[11] It has also been demonstrated that students who adopt a deep approach to learning tend to spend a longer time studying.[11] These levels of processing have been termed the 'learning process complex.'[11]

Research has shown that when students adopt a 'deep approach' to learning they look for meaning in their studies, interact actively with what is being learned, and make real-life links to their studying.[11] They examine evidence critically and use it with caution. They are able to relate new ideas to existing knowledge, and they show interest in what they are learning. Conversely, students who take a 'surface approach' rely on rote learning, and restrict their learning to the syllabus and specific tasks. They lack self-confidence and are anxious about assessment requirements. They fail to make links between ideas and are fact driven. These are not innate characteristics of students, but rather a response to a situation.

It is desirable for structured 'deep learning' to be encouraged within higher education, as this will enable students to take responsibility for and become 'active' participants in their own learning.[13] Reflection on and analysis of experience and practice will also be a key element of this type of learning. Use of case study can help to facilitate this process.

It has been suggested that learning is context dependent.[11] Certainly the learning environment, rigid assessment techniques, interpersonal student–teacher relationships and lack of choice with regard to content and method are vital factors to consider when looking at the quality of learning. The creation of a nurturing environment that supports and challenges the student needs to be considered. Students should be challenged to develop the various skills that are required in order to become a critical thinker. However, this must be done within a supportive environment that is conducive to the ethos of learning.[14] The teacher, when using a case study, should be aware of his or her own facilitative skills in the process of ensuring a creative environment.

The disadvantages of case study

The disadvantages of case study are that attention needs to be given to establishing clear learning objectives, a good structure is required to ensure realism, and plenty of preparation time is needed.[3] Clarity is essential when generating case studies. This is why it is often helpful to use 'real-life' examples. However, the utilisation of such real-life situations has the potential to cause difficulties with regard to confidentiality.[5]

To counter this, an innovative way of using case study is to allow the students to explore their experience and creativity by devising their own case studies. This method may avoid the possibility of breaching confidentiality, as it is a group exercise that includes each individual's input, experience, thoughts and feelings. This was demonstrated in a session in which students were asked to create case studies following an interactive lecture that explored the issues of adherence and compliance in the healthcare setting. Although appropriate case studies were produced by most of the groups, one was a rather extreme example. This created some difficulties for the group that, following the exchange of case studies, was given the extreme example. The difficulties arose as they attempted to address the issues raised and find solutions.

It could be argued that a disadvantage of student-centred learning is that less material is covered, as more time is required for the process to occur. This might be true, but if we are encouraging deeper learning then it is more important to explore as many concepts and avenues as possible within the given time than to attend to every detail, which students can research for themselves.

Some of the literature argues that case studies do not result in true experiential learning. However, they do share many of the common concepts – for example, student-centredness, interaction, a degree of autonomy, and face-to-face confrontation. Interpersonal and negotiation skills are needed in order to find one's place within the group according to one's preferred learning style. Research into nurse teachers' attitudes to experiential learning has found a wide variety of thoughts and feelings.[2] The suggestion that it could be likened to 'doing therapy' concurred with arguments by Rogers and Heron (both cited by Quinn[2]). Blending the two in an educational setting has both ethical and moral implications. Using case studies may involve a demand for a more 'humanist' teacher, who attends to the needs of the students as well as the subject matter.[3] In my opinion it is important to strike a balance here – we have to consider students as individuals. Certainly we often do need to have very humanist skills at our fingertips to help to give guidance on academic and pastoral dilemmas. However, we also need to be aware of professional boundaries and not become immersed in students' problems. The classroom is not an appropriate setting in which to 'do therapy', and as teachers we are not in a suitable position to do so.

Summary

It can be seen that, as with all learning and teaching strategies, there are advantages and disadvantages to the use and scope of case study. The use of case study enables the session to be student focused, although it must be remembered that individual learning styles will need to be scrutinised in order to assess the usefulness of this method to the group in question. Case study can be a tool for reflection, which in turn helps to build expertise in the safety of the individual's own private space or within clinical supervision.

However, when case studies are created, confidentiality must be maintained, as clients/patients may be easily identifiable. Although case study may not be considered by some to be true experiential learning, it is a useful tool to explore as a learning and teaching strategy. It is important to be aware of the implications of teachers entering into a 'therapy' situation, in order to avoid ethical and moral dilemmas.

□ Case study is a useful tool for examining and exploring previous and future practice.

□ This method promotes cooperation and collaboration.

□ Thoughts, feelings, behaviours and attitudes can be assessed.

□ Case study enhances reflection and deeper learning.

□ Case studies may take time to create, and if drawn from 'real life' and/or practice, issues of confidentiality require careful consideration.

References

1 Neary M. *Teaching, Assessing and Evaluation for Clinical Competence: a practical guide for practitioners and teachers.* Cheltenham: Stanley Thornes Publishers Ltd; 2000.

2 Quinn FM. *Principles and Practice of Nurse Education.* 4th ed. Cheltenham: Stanley Thornes Publishers Ltd; 2000.

3 Reece I, Walker S. *Teaching, Training and Learning: a practical guide incorporating FENTO standards.* 5th ed. Sunderland: Business Education Publishers Ltd; 2003.

4 Biggs J. *Teaching for Quality Learning at University.* 2nd ed. Buckingham: Open University Press; 2003.

5 Ross JW, Wright L. Participant-created case studies in professional training. *J Workplace Learn Employee Counsel Today.* 2000; **12:** 23–8.

6 O'Cinneide B. Proposed enhancement of the contribution of the teaching note to the case-writing process. *J Eur Indust Train.* 1998; **22:** 28–32.

7 Jarvis P, Gibson S. The teacher practitioner and mentor: In: *Nursing, Midwifery, Health Visiting and the Social Services.* 2nd ed. Cheltenham: Stanley Thornes Publishers Ltd; 1997.

8 Joel MA, Modell HI. *Active Learning in Secondary and College Science Classrooms: a working model for helping the learner to learn.* Mahwah, NJ: Lawrence Erlbaum Associates Inc.; 2003.

9 Student-centered learning; www.wcer.wisc.edu/step/ep301/Fall2000/Tochonites/stu_cen.html (accessed 14 May 2004).

10 Active learning; www.wcer.wisc.edu/step/ep301/Fall2000/Tochonites/active.html (accessed 14 May 2004).

11 Cowman S. The approaches to learning of student nurses in the Republic of Ireland and Northern Ireland. *J Adv Nurs.* 1998; **28:** 899–910.

12 Wong FKY, Loke AY, Wong M *et al.* An action research study into the development of nurses as reflective practitioners. *J Nurs Educ.* 1997; **36:** 476–81.

13 Lowe PB, Kerr CM. Learning by reflection: the effect on educational outcomes. *J Adv Nurs.* 1998; **27:** 1030–33.

14 Melland HI, Volden CM. A nurturing learning environment – on- or off-line. *Nurs Forum.* 2001; **36:** 23–8.

CHAPTER 6

Reflecting on reflection

Jan Gidman

Introduction

Reflection seems to have been the learning strategy of choice in health and social care since its popularisation in the 1990s. This chapter will consider definitions of reflection, discuss its advantages as a learning and teaching strategy, and critique its widespread adoption in the education of health and social care professionals. It will outline the value of reflection in promoting professional education, but will also acknowledge the difficulties often faced by students and their mentors in using reflection in practice settings, and it will argue that curricula should adopt a spiral approach which integrates theory and practice.

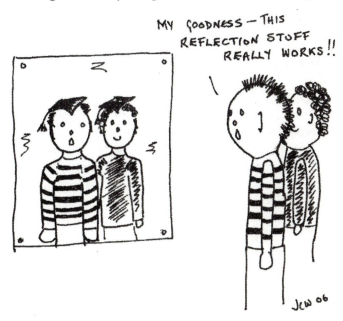

Before writing this chapter, I reflected on my own experience of using reflection, both as a personal learning strategy and to promote learning in students. My initial nurse training was based on anatomy, physiology and symptom management, following the medical model of care. Although 'learning by doing' was a major component of my programme, this was not formalised, and no specific strategies were employed to promote experiential learning or to integrate theory and practice. Many years later, I undertook a post-registration BSc (Hons) in nursing studies, as a part-time student, while working as a night sister. This programme encouraged academic progression, and it focused on the theories underpinning healthcare and the models that had been developed to promote holistic rather than medical care. However, reflection was not incorporated into the programme, and learning from practice occurred in an ad-hoc manner without support from lecturers.

It was when I commenced my postgraduate certificate in education that I first encountered reflection as a strategy to promote experiential learning, and I embraced it wholeheartedly. I used reflection not only within my teaching practice, but also to build up my portfolio to demonstrate professional development. Although I was unaware of it at the time, re-reading some of those accounts identified a major difference in approach to my reflections as a novice teacher and to those as an experienced ward sister. This led me to consider levels of reflection not only in relation to cognitive ability, but also in relation to expertise within professional practice, and to reassess my expectations of students.

I continued my own education by undertaking a Master of Education programme. This allowed me to further develop the level of my reflection and to explore its theoretical and evidence base as a learning and teaching strategy. I became a great advocate of reflection, and have used it to promote experiential learning and the integration of theory and practice with a wide range of students, including pre-registration nursing programmes and post-registration education with health and social care professionals. When I led a level 3, 30-credit module on reflection, I began to question the way that reflection has been adopted wholesale for professional education. Students were telling me that it was only towards the end of the module that they felt truly able to reflect. In addition to this, I had used a phenomenological approach to analyse interview data, as part of a Welsh National Board research project to explore practice-based learning. I interviewed final-year Bachelor of Nursing students and was surprised to discover that although the curriculum explicitly incorporated reflection, students did not articulate this when recounting their experiences of learning in the practice setting.[1] This prompted me to review the value of reflection, and reflective models, in pre-registration education programmes and to consider appropriate levels of reflection in relation to study at an academic level.

Defining reflection

The literature on reflection originates from a range of sources, including education, psychology and sociology, and there appears to be a lack of clarity in the use of terminology between different authors and disciplines – for example, in relation to the terms 'reflection', 'critical reflection', 'reflective practice' and 'reflexivity.' A commonly accepted definition of reflection is that it is:

> the process of creating and clarifying the meaning of experience (present or past) in terms of self (self in relation to self and self in relation to the world). The outcome is changed conceptual perspective.[2]

(p.101)

The interrelationship between reflection and other processes (e.g. cognition, critical thinking, memory, emotion, intuition and imagination) is also unclear at present in relation to learning. Within higher education, it often seems that we have a fragmented view of reflection. However, Moon[3] argues that the apparent differences in reflection are due not to different types of reflection but to differences in the application of the reflective process, and that authors are presenting a range of frameworks for reflection. She proposes what she refers to as a 'common-sense' definition, in that reflection involves the process of learning and the representation of that learning, implies purpose and involves complex mental processing for issues which have no obvious solution.

Freshwater and colleagues[4] distinguish between terms that are sometimes used interchangeably:

- *reflective practice* – thinking about how you practise and developing an awareness of how practice is structured
- *critical reflection* – thinking about how you are thinking about practice and deconstructing practice from a personal perspective
- *reflexivity* – thinking about how you are thinking within the political, ethical, social and historical context from a global perspective.

CASE STUDY 6.1

The findings of my earlier research study[1] were presented and discussed at a practice placement meeting within a local NHS trust. Mentors perceived that, in general, students viewed reflection as a model that they used when completing written assignments, and not one that they applied to practice. They felt that encouraging students to reflect on the experience gained while caring for patients needed greater emphasis. However, they recognised the difficulties involved in actually finding time to do this, because of competing priorities within their roles.

My experience of teaching within higher education has led me to believe that students often find it difficult to progress from reflective practice to critical reflection, and that reflexivity is often only evident at postgraduate level. Case study 6.1 illustrates the difficulties that are often encountered by students and their mentors when trying to use reflection as a learning and teaching strategy in practice settings.

Following this discussion, the clinical practice facilitators decided to pilot student-led reflective sessions in the orthopaedic and rehabilitation units of the trust. The sessions provided a wide variety of topics and themes for discussion and reflection – for example, challenging poor practice, and sharing experiences of critical incidents and how to maximise learning opportunities. Student evaluations have been very positive to date. They felt that the group approach provided opportunities to discuss and compare practice situations and highlighted the fact that peers often experienced similar emotions. It increased the opportunity to reflect on how they would have felt or dealt with learning opportunities that they did not personally encounter. It promoted learning from mistakes and provided the opportunity to openly discuss these topics with a more experienced practitioner in the form of the clinical practice facilitator. Informal discussions with practitioners indicated that the students returned to the clinical areas with renewed confidence and were increasingly proactive in seeking learning opportunities. It is now intended to extend these sessions to other areas, to develop an inter-professional focus and to develop strategies to increase the level of reflection.

Historical perspective and advantages of reflection

Dewey[5] and Habermas[6] are often considered to be the two theorists who provide the underpinnings to reflection as a learning and teaching strategy. Both theorists propose that reflection serves to generate knowledge, but they adopt different philosophical stances and present different frameworks and objectives. Dewey[5] focuses on the process of reflection as a means of making sense of the world and as a means of promoting effective education, whereas Habermas[6] focuses on the place of this process in the acquisition, development and consideration of knowledge as a means of promoting the empowerment of the individual.

Dewey[5] was interested in the nature of reflection and how it occurs. He adopted an educational and psychological approach and based his work on observations of his own learning and that of others. He was concerned with the skills with which we manipulate knowledge and reprocess it towards a purpose, describing the process of reflection as:

> the kind of thinking that consists in turning a subject over in the mind and giving it serious thought.[5]

(p.12)

Dewey proposes that reflection is a cognitive process which involves a chain of linked ideas that are evident as a stream of consciousness. Dewey's theory emphasises perplexity as the stimulus for reflection. He argues that the process is initiated when the individual is faced with situations of uncertainty, doubt or difficulty.

The role of emotion, within the processes of reflection, has been explored by Boud and colleagues,[7] who suggested that this has a major impact on learning for students.

This was certainly evident in my own research project. Several of the respondents in this project described critical incidents with patients. It was evident that they had been emotionally involved in the experiences and it was this emotional response, as well as recognition of a feeling of uncertainty, that had promoted the reflective process. The case study described above also demonstrated that emotion could be used to trigger the reflective process. The clinical practice facilitators involved in the project were aware of students' emotional responses to situations and were able to debrief and support them. However, they were also able to promote learning, not only for the students who were directly involved in the experience, but also for their peers. This has similarities to the clinical supervision process for qualified staff, which is a natural progression from these reflective sessions.

Habermas[6] argues that knowledge needs to be considered within a social, as well as an individual, context. The philosophical stance of Habermas[6] is different from that of Dewey[5] in that he presents reflection as a tool which is used in the development of particular forms of knowledge. He focuses on the nature of the processes that generate these different forms of knowledge, and he describes three knowledge constitutive interests:

- *technical (instrumental) knowledge* – an individual uses this to understand and to gain control over his or her environment. This is particularly applicable to the empirical and analytical sciences, which value the stance of objectivity
- *interpretative knowledge* – an individual uses this form of knowledge to understand behaviour in terms of communication. This involves the interpretation and integration of ideas, and is particularly applicable to the social sciences, which Habermas[6] argues require an additional form of knowledge to that provided within the technical constitutive interest
- *emancipatory interests* – these require the development of knowledge in order to understand self in relation to the human condition and self in context. Habermas argues that this form of knowledge takes account of the personal, social and political contexts and can contribute to the emancipation of social groups.

This focus on the process, as opposed to the product, of learning makes reflection advantageous to professional education, because it encourages practitioners to examine how, why and what they are thinking and feeling during an experience, rather than focusing on the outcome alone.[8] Health and social care programmes have become increasingly outcome- and competency-driven in recent years. However, the personal academic tutor system and the use of reflective portfolios can be used to ensure that the focus on the process of learning is not lost. This is of particular importance in professional programmes, where students need to develop both a lifelong approach to learning and increasing levels of reflection. These programmes should also prepare students for Habermas' highest level of knowledge – emancipatory interests – if they are to influence health and social care.

Barnett[9] contends that Habermas[6] used reflection as a tool to evaluate society, and he argues that higher education requires a state of critical being and not just critical thinking, and that emancipatory reflection enables the empowerment of practitioners to understand their true situations and create the freedoms that they need. This is of great relevance to health and social care practitioners who work within ever changing political and professional contexts. Taylor[8] expands the work of Habermas,[6] developing a theory of reflection based on the three forms of constitutive knowledge interests. She proposes that instrumental knowledge leads to technical reflection, interpretative knowledge leads to practical reflection, and emancipatory knowledge leads to emancipatory reflection.[8] However, there is disagreement in the literature as to whether instrumental knowledge can actually be classified as reflection.

Donald Schön[10,11] is recognised as the leading theorist on reflection as a means to enhance the professions. The main points of his theory were derived from earlier work by Argyris and Schön.[12] Schön[10,11] proposed that practitioners draw on theories-in-use more than they draw on espoused theories. He describes theories-in-use as those context-specific theories that are used by practitioners to guide everyday practice, and espoused theories as the theories that are learned in formal educational settings.

Schön's theory[10,11] describes two main forms of reflection, namely reflection-on-action and reflection-in-action. Reflection-on-action is a fairly narrow concept, is retrospective and may be either verbalised or non-verbalised. In contrast to reflection-on-action, reflection-in-action is situated within the activity itself and is said to occur when there is no obvious action, and it is associated with theories-in-use. Schön argues that reflection-in-action only occurs when an action has potential unexpected consequences. This is consistent with Dewey's notion of perplexity.[5]

Schön[10,11] proposed the use of a virtual world or practicum to allow practitioners to develop in a risk-free environment:

> in the varied topography of professional practice, there is a high, hard ground where practitioners can make effective use of research-based theory and technique, and there is a swampy lowland where situations are confusing 'messes' incapable of technical solution . . . in the swamp are the problems of greatest human concern.[10]

(p.42)

Again, it is apparent that this is of great relevance to the education of health and social care professionals. Students need to develop the ability to respond to a range of complex situations within this swampy lowland. Problem-based learning is a strategy that provides the opportunity for students to explore complex situations within practice by means of hypothetical scenarios. This could also provide the opportunity for lecturers to integrate reflective sessions with information gathering, to explore students' decision-making processes (i.e. to focus on the process as well as the product of learning).

Patricia Benner's theory 'from novice to expert'[13] has also been very influential in the education of healthcare professions, and is widely used to promote and assess the development of skills and competence. Although it is not considered explicitly as a theory of reflection, but rather as one of experiential learning, Benner[13] does articulate the expert but often tacit knowledge that is demonstrated by experienced nurses, and explores the role of intuition in this process. Benner's work was developed from that of Dreyfus and Dreyfus[14] on skill acquisition. Dreyfus and Dreyfus observed airline pilots and proposed that as they became more skilled and experienced they relied less on rules, guidelines and maxims and more on intuition to guide their practice.

Benner[13] describes five stages of development, which she refers to as novice, advanced beginner, competent, proficient and expert. She provides detailed descriptions of the expectations and observable behaviours of practitioners at each of these levels.

1 *Novices* display limited ability to apply knowledge and principles learned in formal educational settings to the reality of practice. At this stage the practitioner is bound very firmly by rules.

2 *Advanced beginners* are able to apply knowledge to a range of practice situations and follow guidelines, which are less restrictive than rules and require some decision making by the individual.

3 *Competent* practitioners can function independently within practice settings, but have limited ability to respond to unexpected events or situations. This is generally accepted to be the level of registration for practitioners, although some authors argue that they may only be advanced beginners at this stage.

4 *Proficient* practitioners have considerable experience and are able to predict potential problems and view situations 'in the round.'

5 *Expert* practitioners have a large repertoire of experience and have an intuitive grasp of the whole situation.

Benner's theory is often applied within a competence framework in professional education programmes. I would also encourage lecturers to consider it in relation to reflecting on the process of developing these increasing levels of competence.

QUESTIONS TO CONSIDER

- How does the 'expert' make decisions about care?
- How does this link with reflection in action?
- How we can we encourage experienced practitioners to explore this process with students?
- How could the group reflective sessions described earlier encourage this?

It is evident in the above discussion of some of the main theories that underpin reflection that it has many potential advantages for the education of health and social care professionals. Reflection addresses the need for practitioners to learn from practice experience and to use uncertainty to prompt learning. It also provides a strategy to address the complexity of practice in the rapidly changing health and social care climate, and to promote the empowerment of individuals.

Potential difficulties of using reflection

My own experience has led me to question the way in which we currently use reflection within health and social care programmes. This chapter will now address a number of potential difficulties that lecturers and practice educators need to consider before adopting reflection wholesale within health and social care education.

I have used reflection, as both a formal and an informal learning and teaching strategy, within a range of professional education programmes. The formal approach, which is apparent in many health and social care curricula, involves introducing students to theories and models of reflection and then providing time and support for them to develop the necessary skills. This often culminates in the submission of written reflective accounts, which form part of the assessment for the module. It is important that we are able to measure the presence and level of reflection if we are formally assessing students' reflective accounts. However, there is currently a lack of reliable methods for assessing whether reflection has taken place, and if it has, at what level.

Practice-based learning is a vital aspect of student learning, and we need to work closely with practice colleagues to maximise this in both undergraduate and postgraduate programmes. The students in the research study described earlier[1] had learned from their experiences with patients, but had not identified this learning as being due to reflection. This was despite the fact that reflection and reflective models were exemplified within the curriculum. This raises questions with regard to the value of models for promoting reflection. In my experience, it is the facilitation skills of lecturers, practice educators and mentors, rather than the model used, that prompt students to move from thinking to reflection and its associated cognitive skills.

Hargreaves[15] argues that the imperative to achieve academically may discourage reflection that is open and honest. Indeed, she suggests that the formal assessment of reflective accounts may act as a barrier to the students' personal growth and integrity. I have similar reservations about using reflection as a means of formal assessment for students, especially within the early stages of their programme. Assessment tends to value the outcome of reflection, rather than developing the process, and students may be tempted to 'play the game' in order to get a good assignment grade, reinforcing accepted professional values and codes rather than truly reflecting on practice.

Lecturers also need to be aware of the power imbalance between themselves and their students. This is particularly evident when the lecturer is responsible for formal assessment of the student. Cotton[16] argues that the discourse of reflection in nursing tends towards inclusiveness, rather than valuing diversity, and that this can lead to political regulation and the devaluing of individuals and groups who do not conform to the dominant discourse. She argues for new conceptualisations of reflection, with an inclusive perspective, to encourage new meanings, interpretations and political positioning. This would seem to be consistent with Habermas' highest level of knowledge, namely emancipatory interests, which may enable future practitioners to influence health and social care rather than conform to existing norms.

QUESTIONS TO CONSIDER

- Which theories of reflection are used to underpin the curriculum?
- How are students prepared to reflect?
- Which, if any, reflective models will be introduced to the students?
- Is the process of reflection or its product of primary importance?
- Is reflection promoted verbally or in written format?
- Are students encouraged to engage in self-reflection, reflection with peers or reflection with an 'expert'?
- Is reflection formally assessed as part of the programme and, if so, how is the level of reflection measured?
- How does the curriculum promote the development of increasing levels of reflection and the associated cognitive abilities?

Conclusion

This chapter has outlined the work of the main theorists who have influenced the way in which we use reflection as a learning and teaching strategy within professional programmes at both undergraduate and postgraduate levels. It has also suggested that reflection has many benefits, in terms of promoting personal and professional development and empowering students to become effective practitioners, within the ever-changing political context of health and social care. Some of the potential difficulties have also been raised, including power issues associated with the discourse of reflection and its formal assessment. The case study explored issues relating to the application of reflection in practice settings, and identified the need for mentors and practice educators to facilitate the progression of students from thinking to reflection, critical reflection and ultimately reflexivity. This requires programmes to be underpinned by reflective theories and to include explicit strategies to apply these theories to student learning in both university and practice settings.

- ❒ Reflection is a valuable learning and teaching strategy, but is not a panacea for professional education.
- ❒ Reflection should focus on the process as well as the product of learning.
- ❒ Curricula should be underpinned by reflective theories.
- ❒ Curricula should develop increasing levels of reflection and promote professional empowerment.
- ❒ Facilitators of reflection need preparation and support.
- ❒ Assessment of reflection has the potential to create 'false' reflections.
- ❒ Lecturers need to be aware of power issues inherent in the discourse of reflection.

References

1 Gidman J. An exploration of students' perceptions of clinical learning. Occasional paper. *Prof Dev J.* 2001; **5:** 15–18.

2 Boyd EM, Fales AW. Reflective learning: key to learning from experience. *J Humanistic Psychol.* 1983; **23:** 99–117.

3 Moon J. *Reflection in Learning and Professional Development.* London: Kogan Page; 1999.

4 Freshwater D, Jasper M, Gilbert A. *Reflective Practice Master Class.* Qualitative Research in Health and Social Care Conference, Bournemouth, 8–11 September, 2003.

5 Dewey J. *How We Think.* Boston, MA: Heath and Co.; 1933.

6 Habermas J. *Knowledge and Human Interests.* London: Heinemann; 1971.

7 Boud D, Keogh R, Walker D. *Reflection: turning experience into learning.* London: Kogan Page; 1985.

8 Taylor B. *Reflective Practice: a guide for nurses and midwives.* Buckingham: Open University Press; 2000.

9 Barnett R. *The Idea of Higher Education.* Buckingham: Open University Press; 1997.

10 Schön D. *Educating the Reflective Practitioner: towards new design for teaching and learning in the professions.* Aldershot: Avebury Academic Publishing; 1987.

11 Schön D. *The Reflective Practitioner: how practitioners think in action.* Aldershot: Avebury Academic Publishing; 1991.

12 Argyris C, Schön D. *Theory in Practice: increasing professional effectiveness.* San Francisco, CA: Jossey-Bass; 1974.

13 Benner P. *From Novice to Expert.* New York: Addison Wesley; 1984.

14 Dreyfus H, Dreyfus S. *Mind Over Machine: the power of human intuition and expertise in the era of the computer.* Oxford: Blackwell; 1986.

15 Hargreaves J. So how do you feel about that? Assessing reflective practice. *Nurs Educ Today.* 2004; **24:** 196–201.

16 Cotton A. Private thoughts in public spheres: issues in reflection and reflective practices in nursing. *J Adv Nurs.* 2001; **36:** 512–19.

CHAPTER 7

Storytelling and narratives: sitting comfortably with learning

Jan Woodhouse

Reflection

When you think of storytelling you will probably, like me, remember story-time from your childhood. I encountered it both pre-school, when I sat rapt listening to the radio, and then through my school years. The narrators took me to imaginary places where I learned some of the values that society expected of me. For example, Aesop's fables and the Brer Rabbit stories illustrated how greed and a quick fix would not ultimately be beneficial to me as a person.

After I left school and embarked on nurse training, the formal aspect of story-telling ceased and was replaced with anecdotes drawn from the clinical experiences of the tutors. These anecdotes were used to illustrate points in a lecture or a debate.

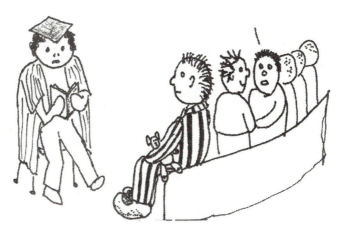

I THINK BARNEY'S REALLY ENJOYING THESE STORYTELLING SESSIONS

JGW 06

They are commonplace in healthcare settings – to be heard in reports, during coffee breaks and wherever healthcare professionals are gathered. These are the 'shop talk', the stories and the narrations of the professions. I participated in them along with everyone else.

Then, several years ago, I undertook a course of study on 'integrative learning', which highlighted the use of storytelling as a teaching strategy. However, this time the focus was not on children but on adults. To illustrate the point, we were read a story about dinosaur characters that charted the differences in and development of the brain. From this I learned that we have a mammalian brain, the limbic brain and the neocortex, each with different functions. Enthused by my encounter with this way of teaching, I was keen to put it into action.

The following week I was teaching 'Reviewing the literature' to a group of post-registered nurses on a research critique module. I rewrote the story of 'Goldilocks and the Three Bears', in the style of a research paper, in order to illustrate that much of research involves an understanding of the terms and jargon of everyday activities. The students seemed appreciative of this approach. Emboldened by this success, a few weeks later I sought to explain 'qualitative research methods' in a similar way. It took me a weekend of thought, writing and refining. I produced a narrative called 'Planet Qualitative' that explained the different approaches to gathering data. This time the outcome of the students' learning was mixed. For quite a few there was puzzlement, as they were unsure of the point of the narrative, while others received the message loud and clear. Months later, however, when the students evaluated the whole of the course, the sessions that were most clearly remembered were those containing the narratives – in the same way that I remember the brain dinosaurs.

When the opportunity has arisen, I have continued to use a limited amount of storytelling. For example, I have delivered sessions on 'breaking bad news' to both medical and nursing students. At the end of the session I read from John Diamond's book *C: because cowards get cancer too*.[1] This is a rich narrative on his experience of being diagnosed with cancer, the receiving of such news and his treatment. I use selected snippets of his story to illustrate the concepts discussed in the session. At the end of the session, the use of John Diamond's story has consistently been positively evaluated by the students.

Defining storytelling

So what is 'storytelling'? And how does it differ from the anecdotes that are already being utilised to illustrate lectures and discussions in the classroom? In order to understand both the concept and the differences, it is necessary to turn first to the early educational literature of the 1980s, in primary and secondary school teaching. They considered the questions 'What is a story? What is the structure of a story? And how does it make a bridge between teaching and learning?' Therefore, in order to explore what we understand by storytelling, like any good storyteller we must start at the beginning, and consider the question 'What is a story?'

Rosen states:

> The story is always out *there* but the important step has still to be taken. The unremitting flow of events must first be selectively attended to, interpreted as holding relationships, causes, motives, feelings, consequences – in a word, *meanings.*[2]
>
> (p.13)

He goes on to say that the story is not enough, but that the telling – the narrative – is important. This notion of telling linked to the word 'narrative' appears to be referring to the process of talking aloud. Kearney reinforces this view:

> all narrative involves . . . a speaker, someone to whom they are speaking and a statement about something (a world, real or imaginary).[3]
>
> (pp.183–4)

This differs from the later, healthcare-related views of the word 'narrative', which see it as a story, which can be either spoken or written.[4-6]

Rosen expands on his definition of a story by adding:

> it is an outcome of a mental process which enables us to excise from our experience a meaningful sequence.[2]
>
> (p.13)

However, it does not stop there, for he further suggests that storytelling has a distinct structure that distinguishes it from normal conversation. This structure has three elements – the story (either real or imagined), the narrative (telling the events) and the narrating (the way that the story is told). This is a familiar model that resonates with the childhood experience described at the beginning of this chapter. The vocalisation of stories is an important factor in the transmission of information, and it is not enough simply to read a story. A spoken narrative is different from a written narrative for, as Rosen's wife comments:

> the printed text of any talk wipes out all speech rhythms, tone, pitch, variation of pace, all eye contact, actions, gestures, mannerisms, physical jerks, quirks, twitches, fleeting grins, frowns, gleams, glares. Indeed, it strikes out completely that entire enigmatic, dynamic container of infinite mysteries – the visible human form.[7]
>
> (p.70)

She considers that the nature of being human is that we are steeped in the oral tradition rather than the written one, and as such it is the spoken word that is the 'main source of inspiration to a whole class.' Here she is talking about teaching children, and it could be debated whether as a strategy for teaching adults, who may be more sceptical and less susceptible to inspiration, its impact could be diminished.

A further contribution to an appreciation of storytelling is provided by the work of Livo and Rietz,[8] who have also commented on its structure. They point out that there are features that distinguish a story. The structure of the story usually begins with an introduction to the setting and characters, in which there is an event, or a series of events, with details, from which a problem is identified. Subsequent events, which occur in a logical sequence to the introduction, are aimed at resolution of the problem, although these events may create other problems. There comes a point in the story where there is resolution or problem solution. There may be a conclusion and finally, although not always, there may be a moral to the story. This provides a story map.[8]

This map may be embellished by use of the voice, movement and other para-linguistic characteristics. Livo and Rietz suggest that mapping enables framing or schemata to form in the memory. Storytelling then becomes:

> a problem-solving activity in which the teller must transform abstract memories for story grammar, language, paralanguage and story content into an integrated, whole, concrete, palpable surface product.[8]

(p.37)

Without this mapping the story would be difficult to tell – the story gets lost in the telling because events are out of sequence or there is no resolution to the problem.

This model of storytelling is recognisable because we all know if we have interrupted someone who is telling a story to a group rather than just having a general conversation. Usually the narrator will return to the story after the interruption has been dealt with. Similarly, we have encountered people who are natural storytellers. They appear to subconsciously adhere to this mapping. Equally, we can think of others who may initially engage us but who leave the audience 'stranded', wondering what was the point of the story. This may explain why the research students seemed puzzled by my story of 'Planet Qualitative' – because the problem-solving aspect was not narrated (a deliberate but wrong move on my part) until about 30 minutes later.

An additional factor to the mapping of stories is that we have a familiar notion of the characters or archetypes contained within the story – a hero or heroine, a younger person, a fool, an old person, a mistreated person, an uncaring person or an evil person. Through these individuals we explore our behaviours and understanding of the 'basic human needs – love, security, understanding, acceptance, success, community and companionship, happiness, knowledge.'[8] These are recognisable components in storytelling that are familiar to us all, for we have all grown up with stories. However, this oral tradition has the potential to disappear, for it has been noted that the media tends to replace storytelling with information.[3]

One could argue that this is the way forward – to expose students to information and let them acquire some learning by some means or another. However, it has already been mentioned that the features of the spoken narrative contain both verbal and non-verbal cues of communication. As both listener to and observer of the storyteller we are therefore picking up on more than the story. Consequently, storytelling has been used in adult education, and palaeontology, geology, the idea of fetal development and chemical reaction have been cited as sciences that transmit their knowledge through the use of storytelling.[2] It has been suggested that there are four scales which provide a bridge between narrative and learning:

1 the *scale of spontaneity* or the degree of improvisation – from a traditional tale to a spur-of-the-moment blurting out

2 the *scale of fictiveness* or the degree to which the events are invented – from fantasy to true story

3 the *scale of embeddedness* or the degree to which the story stands on its own – from telling a story to fulfil a storytelling requirement to providing a story at an ad-hoc moment

4 the *scale of economy* or how much is left to the hearer – from the sparsest story to a fully elaborated version.[2]

(p.17)

Considering stories in healthcare in relation to this model, I would suggest that most of them are true, short, spontaneous anecdotes which are rarely planned. What this model offers us is the chance to explore and use storytelling in healthcare to a greater degree and purpose. Thus we could use a planned element around a long, fictitious or traditional tale, for example, when using storytelling as a teaching strategy. This may cause the teacher to consider the question 'What type of story should I use in this planned element?'

In medical education, it has been suggested that four types of stories are used, namely clinical imagination, exploring 'otherness', stories as a research tool and critical reflection on practice.[9] As a research tool, stories are recognised in the guise of 'narratives.' They aid inquiry into areas such as the exploration of male sexuality,[10] nursing student experiences,[6,11,12] management issues[13] and the lives of centenarians.[14] Reflections on nursing practice and patients' narratives have been explored by Koenig and Zorn,[15] who propose that the types of stories that emerge are those of illness, crisis and transition. Additional types of stories that are common in nurse education include 'real stories' (or case studies), 'true stories' (which do not use events involving real people) and 'hypothetical stories' (such as a made-up scenario).[16] It has been observed that students prefer real or true stories rather than hypothetical ones.[16] It is only possible to speculate as to why this might be so. However, what emerges is that storytelling is of use to healthcare education.

The advantages of storytelling

Using the keyword 'storytelling' to explore the literature in the traditional healthcare education texts did not yield many results. More success was achieved using the keyword 'narrative.' Perhaps this is because storytelling is considered to be a pedagogical strategy as opposed to an androgogical one. Perhaps adults feel more comfortable with the term 'narrative' than with 'storytelling', which resonates with childhood. Whichever word is used, it is suggested that there are many positive benefits of utilising it as a teaching strategy.

First, as I found, it gains the students' attention.[15–19] It enables the students to be exposed perhaps to a moral dilemma[16] or a problem-solving exercise.[17,20] Students can use storytelling to share stories of success and develop a sense of community.[15] They can also use it to explore personal roles and make sense of their lives.[19] Davis[21] suggests that in children, if they write stories using the third person, storytelling allows honest expression as they project themselves into the fictitious characters. However, healthcare educators[16,22] have proposed that the first person is used, so that students see a story from the perspective of one of the characters. This calls for the use of imagination and concentrates the mind.[16] It may be that the use of imagination enables stories to be remembered,[18,19] like the ones that I and my students recalled. It has also been suggested that storytelling enhances critical thinking,[11,15,19] – an attribute that is much sought in today's healthcare professionals.

The subject for which this strategy appears to be most appropriate is that of developing language.[2,7,23,24] This may be why it is used more frequently in primary and secondary schools than in adult education, where language is already established. However, Leight[23] points out that nursing and other healthcare professions have two languages – scientific and observational – and consequently storytelling is appropriate, allowing for creative expression and an intuitive application of knowledge. Yet it is not just an understanding of words that is enhanced – storytelling also develops verbal skills.[25] Therefore when I used the story of Goldilocks to express the language of research, this was an appropriate strategy. I was moving the students' language from the familiar to the unfamiliar, or 'from easy to difficult, from simple to complex.'[20]

Other areas that may seem complex for students to understand include ethics and caring – subjects which are emotionally laden. Vella[20] has proposed that listeners experience vicariously the pain and fear of the storyteller. Perhaps this explains the positive response to John Diamond's story. This insight may be achieved through visualisation,[19] and clues as to how the student behaves, together with their coping mechanisms, may also be identified through their recalling of their stories.[15] Certainly storytelling has been used as a therapy for individuals[26] when it has empowered them to voice their personal experiences – for example, working through death, dying and grief in a safe manner. Although it is not the intention to use the classroom as a therapy session, some students do use sessions to discuss difficulties that they have encountered in practice.

One final aspect of storytelling is the interaction that it generates. Fry and colleagues[27] have proposed that teaching is about facilitation, and that exchanging stories allows the teacher to hear the students' perspectives. Similarly, it has been claimed that the process of listening shows respect to others,[20] that it develops relationships,[15] and that the teacher can assess the students at the same time.[15] These positive findings suggest that the benefits of storytelling must be set against the drawbacks in order to evaluate it as a teaching strategy.

The disadvantages of storytelling

The main drawback of using storytelling is that it may take some time to implement,[7,11] and this mirrors my own experience of spending a whole weekend working on one story. Davis[17] also advises against using long stories, although Rosen[7] has reported a storytelling episode that took up 45 minutes of a 70-minute session. However, her sphere of education involves children, and it may be more appropriate to use shorter stories with adults.

Another point to bear in mind is who does the reading. Should it be the lecturer or the student? If it is the latter, this might cause problems, as it has been pointed out that it may not suit the learning style of the student, and it has been observed that some students seem reticent about reading their stories aloud.[19] This may be because the students lack the confidence to read out loud. It has also been pointed out that storytelling requires a safe environment for the students.[19] This notion of safety is highlighted by Fairburn,[16] who uses storytelling as a way of exploring morality and ethics in healthcare. He points out that it demands a lot from students and that his subject matter can seem threatening, as it challenges students' values and may cause them to feel uncomfortable. Therefore it requires trust and a good relationship with the lecturer.[28] In addition, if students are writing their own stories, they may lack self-direction. This aspect has been commented upon by Cooper,[22] who incorporated story writing into an academic assignment. He found that some students found this difficult and would have preferred to have been given a title to work to. This comment suggests that some adult students are not self-directed, and that the diversity of students must be considered when considering teaching styles.

One additional drawback of storytelling may not be related to the students but to the lecturer. Weimer[18] points out that a teacher is an entertainer, and that consequently they should monitor their own motives for storytelling in the first place. This statement rings true. Did *my* preference for using storytelling with the research students override an analysis of other, more suitable approaches? An analysis of my own learning style[29] revealed that I have a strong preference for the visual mode, using images that are either real (e.g. diagrams or charts) or imagined. It is therefore understandable that I might be drawn to a teaching strategy such as storytelling, which requires thoughts to be represented symbolically.[30]

Summary

In summary, storytelling has distinct features with regard to its construction. It is different from the mere written word, allowing for different emphasis to be made during the telling. The interpretation of 'narrative' appears to have changed since the 1980s. There are many different types of story, and it is not possible to recommend one type as being more suitable for a particular subject in healthcare compared with another. There are positive advantages to the use of storytelling in adult education, such as gaining attention, the use of imagination, enabling retention of information and promoting critical thinking. On the other hand, storytelling has its limitations, and its use should be kept within a suitable time frame. It should be recognised that it may not suit the individual learning style of the student, and care and consideration should be given to the subject matter that the story is trying to convey. The preferred teaching style of the lecturer also needs to be included in the equation.

Storytelling is an appropriate tool to use in situations where the development of language, such as the technical terms that are used in the healthcare professions, is required. In addition, it allows the exploration of the meaning of experiences, including those encountered on a daily basis in healthcare, such as illness, death and dying.

Storytelling can be used as a research tool to identify the archetypes that exist in the healthcare setting. In addition, it could be used as an alternative to the traditional academic essay, as an assessment tool to measure the level of learning that the student has attained,[20] or as a measure of competence.[31]

It has been pointed out that storytelling gives meaning to our lives beyond the technological age.[8] It has also been reported that its use increases students' enjoyment of literature, improves their speaking and listening skills, contributes to the development of reading and writing skills, and aids creative thinking.[8] Livo and Reitz have emphasised that students are learning to think creatively:

> creative thinking derives from their ability not only to look, but to see; not only to hear, but to listen; not only to imitate, but to innovate; not only to observe, but to experience the excitement of fresh perception.[8]

> (p.348)

Surely every teacher aspires to this. It is important for the teacher to recognise that storytelling goes on regardless of whether it is planned as a teaching strategy or not. It may be in the form of anecdotes,[15] reflection[22] or a journal,[5] rather than the traditional tales described by Rosen.[7] Whichever mode is used, it continues the tradition of passing on a story, and with it the knowledge acquired by exposure to an experience.

- ❐ Storytelling is a useful teaching strategy for language development and exploring meanings of experiences.
- ❐ It promotes listening, the use of imagination and critical thinking skills.
- ❐ It can also be used to promote writing and verbal skills.
- ❐ Consideration needs to be given to the length of time for which it is used.
- ❐ Storytelling continues the use of the oral tradition.

References

1 Diamond J. *C: because cowards get cancer too.* London: Vermillion; 1998.

2 Rosen H. *Stories and Meanings*. Sheffield: National Association for the Teaching of English; 1985.

3 Kearney R. The crisis of narrative in contemporary culture. *Metaphilosophy*. 1997; **28:** 183–95.

4 Cooper NJ. The use of narrative in the development of critical thinking. *Nurs Educ Today*. 2000; **20:** 513–18.

5 Schaefer KM. Reflections on caring narratives: enhancing patterns of knowing. *Nurs Educ Perspect*. 2002; **23:** 286–93.

6 Ironside PM. Trying something new: implementing and evaluating narrative pedagogy using a multi-method approach. *Nurs Educ Perspect*. 2003; **24:** 122–8.

7 Rosen B. *And None of it was Nonsense: the power of storytelling in school*. London: Mary Glasgow Publications Ltd; 1988.

8 Livo NJ, Rietz SA. *Storytelling: process and practice*. Littleton, CO: Colorado Libraries Unlimited, Inc.; 1986.

9 Greenhalgh T. Storytelling should be targeted where it is known to have greatest added value. *Med Educ*. 2001; **35:** 818–19.

10 Marsiglio W. Making males mindful of their sexual and procreative identities: using self-narrative in field settings. *Perspect Sex Reprod Health*. 2003; **35:** 229–33.

11 Andrews CA, Ironside PM, Nosek C *et al*. Enacting narrative pedagogy: the lived experiences of students and teachers. *Nurs Ed Perspect*. 2001; **22:** 252–9.

12 Spouse J. *Professional Learning in Nursing*. Oxford: Blackwell Publishing; 2003.

13 Fleming D. Narrative leadership: using the power of stories. *Strategy Leadership*. 2001; **29:** 34–5.

14 Mills TL. Listening from the sidelines: the telling and retelling of stories by centenarians. *Generations*. 2003; **27:** 16–20.

15 Koenig JM, Zorn CR. Using storytelling as an approach to teaching and learning with diverse students. *J Nurs*. 2002; **41:** 393–9.

16 Fairburn GJ. Ethics, empathy and storytelling in professional development. *Learn Health Soc Care*. 2002; **1:** 22–32.

17 Davis BG. *Tools for Teaching*. San Francisco, CA: Jossey-Bass; 1993.

18 Weimer M. *Learner-Centred Teaching: five key changes to practice*. San Francisco, CA: John Wiley & Sons; 2002.

19 Davidson MR. A phenomenological evaluation: using storytelling as a primary teaching method. *Nurs Educ Pract*. 2003: **3:** 1–6.

20 Vella JK. *Learning to Listen, Learning to Teach: the power of dialogue in educating adults*. San Francisco, CA: Jossey-Bass; 2002.

21 Davis P. Attitudes to reading: what can stories tell us? *Reading*. 1998; **November issue:** 12–15.

22 Cooper NJ. The use of narrative in the development of critical thinking. *Nurs Educ Today*. 2000; **20:** 513–18.

23 Leight SB. Starry night: using stories to inform aesthetic knowing in women's health nursing. *J Adv Nurs*. 2002; **37:** 108–14.

24 Muñoz ML, Gillam RB, Peña ED *et al*. Measures of language development in fictional narratives of Latino children. *Language Speech Hear Serv Schools*. 2003; **34:** 332–42.

25 Waller A, O'Mara DA, Tait L *et al.* Using written stories to support the use of narrative in conversational interactions: case study. *Augment Altern Communication.* 2001; **17**: 221–32.

26 McArdle S, Byrt R. Fiction, poetry and mental health: expressive and therapeutic uses of literature. *J Psychiatry Ment Health Nurs.* 2001; **8**: 517–24.

27 Fry H, Ketteridge S, Marshall S. *A Handbook for Teaching and Learning in Higher Education.* London: Kogan Page; 2003.

28 Clarke A, Hanson EJ, Ross H. Seeing the person behind the patient: enhancing the care of older people using a biographical approach. *J Clin Nurs.* 2003; **12**: 697–706.

29 North Carolina State University. *Learning Styles*; www.engr.ncsu.edu (accessed 13 February 2004).

30 Ryokai K, Vaucelle C, Cassell J. Virtual peers as partners in storytelling and literacy learning. *J Comput Assist Learn.* 2003; **19**: 195–208.

31 Hargreaves J, Lane D. Delya's story: from expert to novice, a critique of Benner's concept of context in the development of expert nursing practice. *Int J Nurs Stud.* 2001; **38**: 389–94.

CHAPTER 8

Role play: a stage of learning

Jan Woodhouse

Reflection

I played my first role when I was four years old. I was cast as an angel in the church nativity play. One of my fellow 'angels' accidentally (or maybe deliberately) tipped my cardboard halo askew, and I reckon that I have never been the same since! At junior school we were encouraged to write and act out our own plays, and a box of costumes and props helped to facilitate this process. However, at secondary school any potential acting career that I might have had ground to a halt when I was turned down for a part in the school production of Oscar Wilde's *The Importance of Being*

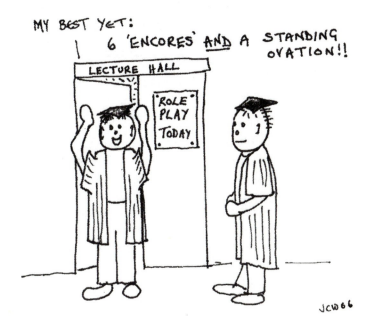

Earnest. The opportunity to act did not occur again until I started my nursing career, only it didn't feel like acting as I had previously known it (except during hospital pantomime productions).

I can recall 'playing a patient' as my fellow students practised bed-making, bandaging, administering a medicine (in reality the 'medicine' was a chocolate sweet, which provided an added incentive to be the patient!) and various other non-invasive, tasks. These activities, which were undertaken in a semi-serious fashion, gave me an insight into how a patient might feel under similar circumstances. There was one particularly powerful moment when the tutor came in and announced (in role) that he had been sent by the local mental health unit with instructions to detain us for the next 48 hours. He asked us individually for our responses. Mine was to question the decision, while others stated that they would fight anyone – either verbally or physically – who tried to drag them away from their home. The tutor then came out of role and asked us to consider how our responses might mirror those of patients detained under the Mental Health Act.

The notion of acting in a role has not been confined to the classroom, and through my formative professional career I have played out roles in practice – acting confident when I felt insecure, acting calm when I felt panicky, acting forceful when my natural inclination is to liberalism. These acted roles end up as a professional identity, and eventually it becomes difficult to know where one stops and the other begins.

While gaining a professional identity I have encountered role play many times, and have played a variety of roles, such as patient, client, student, team member, counsellor and healthcare professional. I have always enjoyed participating in this teaching strategy, but I recognise that this is not true for everybody, and that the very mention of role play can cause students to look in the opposite direction or, even worse, can bring them out in a cold sweat of anxiety and fear.

Therefore the challenge for anyone using role play as a teaching strategy in healthcare education is to maximise learning and promote the acquiring of skills and professional identity, while at the same time minimising the negative effect that this teaching strategy might have on the student.

Definition

So what is meant by role play? I have discussed acting, plays and aspects of experiential exercises within my reflection. A number of texts[1-3] comment on our understanding of the term 'role' (i.e. that we each have many roles in our life, such as parent, partner, child, etc.) before going on to define role play. Within healthcare there are also numerous roles, such as doctor, nurse, therapist, patient, client, administrator, secretary, and so on. Often there may be issues of power accompanying these roles and aspects of social position.[1] In addition, we may be helped in these roles by props such as uniforms, artefacts such as stethoscopes and, of course, language. One only has to look at cartoons that represent the professions to realise that society carries around with it cognitive images of the props of roles – so doctors stereotypically wear white coats and nurses wear short uniforms and caps. However, the purpose of role play is often to get away from these stereotypical images.[3] Once we have an understanding of the term 'role', we can then move on to what is meant by role play.

According to van Ments,[1] role play is 'a type of communication.' It is a form of communication that is simulation, not reality,[4] and it is 'one particular type of simulation that focuses attention on the interaction of people with one another.'[1] Sogorno brings together the concepts of role and role play, and provides the following definition:

> a learning activity in which participants act out a set of defined role behaviors (*sic*) or position with a view to acquiring desired experiences. A role-playing scenario could be mimicking, demonstrative or illustrative of specific concepts, problems or situations.[5]

> (p.356)

In addition, unlike drama, the essence of role play is that it is unrehearsed and that the players act spontaneously.[6] So according to these definitions my youthful experiences were of drama, while those that I encountered in healthcare education were role-play situations.

Within role play, students can be themselves or another person, where they are asked to behave exactly as they feel that a particular person would.[1] However, the role player is not confined to the students, and the tutor may be a participant, a position that is known as 'teacher-in-role.'[7] Alternatively, other staff, clinicians,[8] practitioners[9] or actors[10] may be brought in to be players. Whoever the role player is, there is adoption of a role of social position (e.g. doctor, nurse, manager, patient, worker), and these roles are set in a context (e.g. home, hospital, GP surgery), to which is added the function or purpose of the individuals being there.

Thus the student is presented with a scenario consisting of these elements – role, context, and function or purpose. The aim of the role player, within the given scenario, 'is to feel, react and behave as closely as possible to the way someone placed in that particular situation would do.'[1] In order for this to occur there has to be a supportive learning environment, and one way of achieving this is by paying heed to the way in which role play is implemented as a teaching strategy.

Implementing role play

It is important to remember the initial emotional response to the words 'role play' – some students may baulk at the very mention of it. Pulsford[13] suggests that you can actually use role play to find out the feelings of students about role play! The idea behind this approach is that the students can explore the topic, discovering for themselves those conditions that facilitate role play as a teaching strategy and those aspects that become barriers. Each student, within the role play, has an opportunity to air their attitudes and experiences either as 'themselves' or in their role of 'student for role play' or 'student against role play.'

Whatever method is used to introduce the strategy, the tutor must ensure that there is a structured process that aims to minimise 'problems and negative learning.'[11] Therefore careful planning is required before embarking on the use of role play (*see* Box. 8.1).

BOX 8.1 Strategies for the implementation of role play

- Establish a supportive relationship.
- Provide a clear rationale for its use.
- Identify objectives for the experience.
- Brief the group on the process and objectives.
- Provide the students with a time frame.
- Ensure that the participants are voluntary.
- Provide an opt-out clause.
- Monitor the role-play process, class and reactions.
- Relate role play to theoretical concepts.
- Make the link between real life and work.
- Delineate grading criteria (*this is only applicable if the exercise is an assignment*).
- Indicate the role of the observers.
- Facilitate constructive analysis.
- Have a thorough debriefing (both group and individual).
- 'Check out' any individuals who opt out or leave the room.
- Emphasise positive behaviour and avoid criticising individuals.

(Adapted from Northcott,[4] Shearer and Davidhizar,[11] Tolan and Lendrum[12] and Pulsford.[13])

Tolan and Lendrum have suggested that when the tutor gives their rationale for the use of role play, they should not be heavy-handed or spend too long on preparation, as students need to be allowed time to emotionally engage with the scenario rather than become anxious about their role.[12] However, other authors have suggested that students should be given time to consider whether they want to participate, the most frequent timescale mentioned being a week's notice.[8,14,15] I have used both time frames – the short one when I have been teacher-in-role and a long one when the students are to be videoed.

I would also add the rider that if, as a new teacher, you have not used role play before, you should observe an experienced tutor (or become involved as a role player yourself) before embarking on it as a teaching strategy. This will give you a clearer insight into the advantages and disadvantages of the strategy.

Advantages of role play

The first advantage that can be cited is that of familiarity, because of the use of drama in schools.[16] van Ments reports that role play is 'used in schools, colleges, youth clubs, industrial training, health and social care',[1] so there might even be an expectation by students that they will encounter its use within any curriculum. Students have been reported to find role play exciting and challenging,[12] and educators have found it to be a powerful teaching technique.[1]

This potency may be the reason why role play is so widely used, as 'it can be used for messages, expressing or arousing emotion, negotiation and persuasion, or for a variety of other purposes.'[1] Thus it can be seen to be targeting the affective domain. Tolan and Lendrum[12] propose that, in addition to accessing the emotional domain, role play also addresses the cognitive and behavioural domains. So there is an expectation among educationalists that role play may alter attitudes and behaviours,[4,5] both of which are vital aspects of healthcare education, for such change offers alternative ways of dealing with situations.[5]

A further advantage of role play is its versatility. The situations or scenarios can be simple or elaborate, familiar or strange.[1] They can last for a day or for minutes.[1,4] Students can learn by participation (first hand) or through observation (vicarious).[1] Role play can be used to practise telephone conversations,[9] or it can be recorded to provide feedback to participants.[8] For these purposes, recording equipment will be required, using either audio or video equipment. Ashmore and Banks[8] have reported on the interaction of students with 'patients' during role-play sessions. These interactions were audiotaped, and the tapes were then analysed using Heron's six-category intervention framework, looking for signs of catalytic, prescriptive, supportive, informative, confronting or cathartic interactions (as cited in Ashmore and Banks[8]).

Similarly, an entire role play can be videoed, allowing the role players to view themselves and prompting further debate. Although students may express anxiety and reluctance about appearing in front of a camera, the reality is that they soon forget that the camera is there.[15] Feedback gained from video recordings made during role play is a valuable tool for personal development, as is illustrated in the following case study.

CASE STUDY 8.1

I used role play with a group of nursing students in order to illustrate how leaders emerge from a group. The group was videoed as they performed a task. The role players had to assemble a model, using toy bricks, by copying a completed model that was difficult to see. Instructions were soon flying from the viewers of the completed model to the little band of constructors. During the exercise one individual was repeatedly ignored by the group. I considered that the reason for this might have been due to several differences between that participant and the rest of the group (the individual concerned was of a different gender and race, and held strong religious views). The replay of the video allowed me to point out in a constructive way how this individual's contribution to the group task was being sidelined. I was pleased to note, several weeks later, that there had been a shift in the group dynamics and that the individual concerned had moved to a more central position within the group.

More recently role play has been used in online chat discussions,[17] with students taking on different roles and undertaking shared reading of transcripts. It has been noted that this method, which is similar to the classroom situation, also requires moderation by course facilitators.[17]

Perhaps the greatest advantage of role play lies in its contribution to the learning experience. Tolan and Lendrum have commented that role play is able to 'stimulate the imagination and enable course members to engage with people's concerns and complexities within a supportive environment.'[12] They go on to point out that being observed as a role player 'highlights the differences between how people *think* they are communicating and how their communication is perceived by others.'[12] This aspect of communication is important in healthcare, where a large proportion of our daily work involves trying to achieve successful communication with patients, clients, relatives, and other healthcare workers. Using role play as a teaching strategy allows the student to test out their repertoire of behaviours, or to study the interacting behaviours of the group, and helps them to 'to cope with the idea of uncertainty.'[1]

It has already been noted that participation in role play may not be confined to students, as this teaching strategy also provides an opportunity for the tutor to take part as teacher-in-role. It is suggested[1] that if the tutor is playing teacher-in-role then they should use some kind of prop, such as clothing or an artefact, to indicate when they are in role and when they are not. I have played teacher-in-role on many occasions – for example, as a 'manager' or 'interviewee' when role playing mock interviews designed to raise issues concerning the real interview for the student's first professional post. Another example has been as 'the healthcare professional' talking to someone who is about to be given bad news. The latter example enables the transmission of knowledge by role modelling for, as Tolan and Lendrum[12] have pointed out, 'tutors are most effective when they model those skills and attributes which they are advocating.' Box 8.2 lists some of the skills and attributes that may be enhanced by the strategy of role play.

BOX 8.2 Advantages of role play

- It enhances communication.
- It demonstrates how people interact.
- It highlights stereotyping.
- It can be used to explore deep personal blocks and emotions.
- It improves interpersonal skills.
- It can be used with individuals or in group situations.
- It increases empathy.
- Students may become more aware of their own emotions.
- It helps to identify emotions in others.
- It helps individuals to learn to accept both their own feelings and those of others.
- It develops a vocabulary with which to communicate feelings and emotions.
- It may help students to separate their own feelings from those of others.

- It may identify unethical practice.
- It helps students to deal with difficult situations, such as suicide and breaking bad news.
- It develops confidence and self-efficacy.
- It develops cultural competence.
- It is useful for a range of topics, including interviewing, counselling skills, personal relationships, teamworking (e.g. the multi-disciplinary team), leadership and cultural studies.

(Adapted from van Ments,[1] Goldenberg et al.,[6] Hemmingway and Lees,[9] Shearer and Davidhizar,[11] Tolan and Lendrum[12] and Shankar et al.[18])

Disadvantages of role play

It has already been mentioned that students may react negatively to the mere prospect of being involved in a role-play situation. McHardy and Allan[15] have reported that 44% of students have negative feelings about the use of role play, with a further 29% 'sitting on the fence' (i.e. they make up their minds after the experience). Thus the tutor may be faced with the need to 'sell' the idea to the group. One strategy, adopted by Pulsford,[13] has been to use role play to discuss role play, in order to explore the emotional barriers that may be raised by the students. Barriers to a teaching strategy are an important factor in the learning environment, and the wise teacher will take note of them and monitor how the group responds to suggested activities.

For this reason, role play is 'less "safe" than didactic methods',[12] as there is less control, as far as the teacher is concerned, over what occurs during the role play. One cannot predict the emotional responses of the students, either to the notion of the role play itself or to the content of the role play. Northcott[4] has pointed out that role play may awaken previously subdued or suppressed emotions, such as feelings of fear of failure, being pressurised into doing something one would rather not do, choosing to participate, and feeling unsafe.

The length of time spent in role play may also influence its success or failure. Students may find themselves in role for the whole day – for example, if they are on a management development day – and may find this exhausting. Northcott[4] recommends only taking 5 to 10 minutes for role play, and I would concur with this, although if you are teacher-in-role you may extend this period for yourself, but change over the interactions with different students. For example, I played 'patient' to a small group of mental health students and they took it in turns to carry out an assessment on me, each student taking up the interview where the last one had left off. I stayed in role for 20 minutes, while the students took around 5 minutes each.

Students may become 'stuck', not knowing how to progress, which happened in the example cited above. This may indicate that they have reached the end of their repertoire or knowledge, or that they 'find it difficult to move very far from their own persona.'[7] It has been suggested that if you reach a moment like this you can call 'time out' and ask for comments from the participants or the observers about how to proceed.[10]

It is vital to note that the focus of the role play should remain on the educational aspects, rather than being allowed to slip into psychodrama or sociodrama.[4] For example, Northcott[4] cites a situation where role play was used as a means of 'psychometric' testing on a management course. There was no immediate debriefing, and when it came, it was negative. The participant considered the practice unsettling, unprofessional and unethical. This kind of situation led van Ments[1] to point out that role play can be 'ineffective or dangerous, if using the wrong technique.' This further highlights the need for the tutor to work in an ethical fashion[12] and, whenever possible, to be prepared for the unexpected.

If negative emotions are evoked, they can be dealt with in the debriefing. Similarly, students may experience a role play and not understand the point of it. Therefore, as van Ments points out, the tutor 'may have to spend a lot of time helping the group to appreciate the implications of what has happened.'[1]

Replaying audio or video recordings may help to illustrate points, but here another disadvantage rears its head. If the tutor has used audio or video recording equipment, there are issues of consent, confidentiality, disposal and, of course, being able to use the equipment correctly.[19] I once successfully filmed a group role play and then couldn't manage to tune in the TV in order to play it back. In that particular case the opportunity to give immediate feedback was lost. The use of recording equipment is associated with another possible disadvantage, namely the cost of resources. Such equipment may not be readily available, so this is yet another aspect that requires careful consideration during the planning stage.

Finally, some disadvantages of role play have been noted[12] that relate to the tutor. A tutor may become a 'guru' if the students witness good role modelling, and this could engender feelings of inadequacy among the students.[12] This is hardly the desired learning outcome! Similarly, the tutor may want to be 'loved' by the students and therefore may fail to challenge bad practices that are observed during the role play.[12] One solution to these problems is to utilise co-tutoring and/or peer supervision.

If both the advantages and drawbacks of role play are taken into consideration, this can be an enjoyable, safe and powerful strategy for enhancing learning, especially in healthcare education, where the emphasis is on human interactions and the acquiring of professional roles.

Summary

Role play as a teaching strategy has much to offer healthcare education. It can be used to enhance communication and attitudinal skills, and it provides a platform for discussion. However, it must be used with caution, as some students may view the idea of role play negatively. The tutor's first concern is to promote a supportive environment that will enable students to opt in or out of the strategy. Therefore the tutor must work ethically, and it will also be helpful if he or she empathises with any feelings of discomfort among the students, by acknowledging their fears, anxiety, apprehension and reluctance.[12] The more that role play is used in a safe and ethical way, the more students will come to accept it as a valuable tool for learning, in the knowledge that it will help them to gain confidence in their daily interactions.

- ❑ Role play can provide a powerful learning experience.
- ❑ It involves a high degree of learner participation.
- ❑ A variety of personnel can be role players.
- ❑ Audio and video recordings can be used to provide feedback.
- ❑ Students may feel reluctant to participate.
- ❑ Time should be apportioned for briefing, acting and debriefing.

References

1 van Ments M. *The Effective Use of Role Play: a handbook for teachers and trainers.* London: Kogan Page; 1983.

2 Milroy E. *Role Play: a practical guide.* Aberdeen: Aberdeen University Press; 1982.

3 Jones T, Palmer K. *In Other People's Shoes: the use of role play in personal, social and moral education.* Exeter: Pergamon Educational Productions; 1998.

4 Northcott N. Role play: proceed with caution! *Nurs Educ Pract.* 2002; **2**: 87–91.

5 Sogunro OA. Efficacy of role-playing pedagogy in training leaders: some reflections. *J Manag Dev.* 2004; **23**: 355–71.

6 Goldenberg D, Andrusyszyn M-A, Iwasiw C. The effects of classroom simulation on nursing students' self-efficacy related to health teaching. *J Nurs Educ.* 2005; **44**: 310–14.

7 Somers J. *Drama in the Curriculum.* London: Cassell Educational Ltd; 1994.

8 Ashmore R, Banks D. Student nurses' use of their interpersonal skills within clinical role plays. *Nurs Educ Today.* 2004; **24**: 20–29.

9 Hemmingway S, Lees J. Educating NHS Direct advisors to support the client with mental health problems: using role play as a tool to facilitate skill acquisition. *Nurs Educ Pract.* 2001; **1**: 127–33.

10 Hardoff D, Schonmann S. Training physicians in communication skills with adolescents using teenage actors as simulated patients. *Med Educ.* 2001; **35**: 206–10.

11 Shearer R, Davidhizar R. Using role play to develop cultural competence. *J Nurs Educ.* 2003; **42**: 273–5.

12 Tolan J, Lendrum S. *Case Material and Role Play in Counselling Training.* London: Routledge; 1995.

13 Pulsford D. Reducing the threat: an experiential exercise to introduce role play to student nurses. *Nurs Educ Today.* 1993; **13**: 145–8.

14 Sellers SC. Testing theory through theatrics. *J Nurs Educ.* 2002; **41**: 498–500.

15 McHardy P, Allan T. Closing the gap between what industry needs and what HE provides. *Educ Training.* 2000; **42**: 496–508.

16 Hornbrook D. *Education and Dramatic Art.* 2nd ed. London: Routledge; 1998.

17 Phillips JM. Chat role play as an online strategy. *J Nurs Educ.* 2005; **44**: 43.

18 Shankar PR, Dubey AK, Subish P. Critical evaluation of drug promotion using role plays. *Med Educ.* 2006; **40:** 459–89.

19 Fowler J. The use of video cameras in one college of nursing. *Nurs Educ Today.* 1993; **13:** 66–8.

CHAPTER 9

Creative activities

Jan Woodhouse

Reflection

When I think of the arts and games in the classroom, I am transported back to the days of tins containing poster paints, piles of much-used paint pallets and pots of lumpy glue. Pursuing art as a subject depended on whether the teachers considered your drawing ability was up to scratch. One art teacher was rather scathing about my abilities, but I developed a thick skin and pursued the subject just to spite her. Similarly, music was dependent on individual talent, although I give credit to my secondary school that if you couldn't sing, dance or play an instrument then at least you could learn to appreciate 'the picture' that the classical composers were conveying.

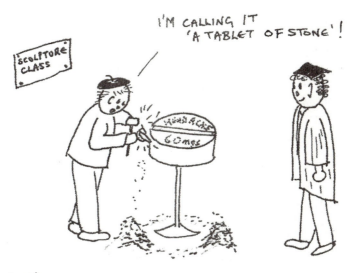

Games (the board versions, rather than physical education) were limited to the end of autumn and summer terms, while the teachers caught up with their marking and report writing. Thus the arts and games were considered to be 'fun' activities and seemed to have little to do with the learning process.

Then in my 'O'-level year I had a new English teacher. He set my class a project. We were divided into groups, and each group had to explore Shakespeare's 'Seven Ages of Man.' My best friend and I had 'Childhood.' The pair of us spent a laughter-filled weekend selecting poems, writing a play, rehearsing it and selecting music to convey the ups and downs of this life stage. I now think that we gave more consideration to the concept of childhood than we could have done in any set essay. What is more we had fun, both in the planning and in the execution of the project.

When I started my basic nurse education I found my 'O' level in art useful, as I was able to draw reasonable reproductions of parts of the body, and encountered many 'draw and label' exercises during sessions on anatomy and physiology. The colours chosen helped to identify the mechanics of the body – red for arteries, blue for veins, yellow for the lymphatic system, green for bile, and brown for . . . the end product of the digestive system.

It wasn't until I started extending my post-registered nurse education that I encountered the arts again. I was on a teaching course and the topic was 'Assessment.' The tutor started this session by inviting us to listen to a piece of music and assess its qualities. I was struck by this use of transference of a concept (assessment) from one medium (music) to another (nursing).

Similarly, I have encountered several games for teaching management concepts (*see* Chapter 11), such as leadership styles and teambuilding. Arts and games used in this way have two things in common – they have an element of fun attached to them, and they result in active learning.

Defining the creative arts

So what is meant by the use of creative art? Taking a philosophical view of the creative arts, Hansen[1] uses the word 'poetics' to denote aesthetics or an art form, and comments that 'it can represent studies of makings, creations and compositions',[1] and as such enables an individual to make sense of the world by considering influences and perceptions. Hansen also suggests that poetics 'highlight truths about human thought and conduct.'[1] Certainly the use of art has revealed human behaviours across the centuries, from the earliest cave drawings to the latest contender for the Turner Prize.

Art is regarded as part of the humanities, a term which implies the use of art, music and literature. The humanities can be defined as 'cultural representation of human experiences',[2] and therefore have an important place in healthcare education. However, their use has been limited, with a reliance on scientific approaches rather than on the creative arts. Perhaps this has been due to the fact that teaching in healthcare education was geared to the medical model, with its corresponding scientific discipline. Nevertheless, experiences and perceptions of the way in which we view the world help us to gain a holistic picture of understanding. Whereas the scientific model brings logicality and description, the humanities model brings emotion and comprehension, and it is the latter two aspects that creative art teaching strategies help to achieve.

Creative art has a plethora of guises and can utilise a variety of media (*see* Box 9.1).

BOX 9.1 Examples of creative activities

- Poetry
- Prose
- Collage
- Sketches and plays
- Photographic essays
- Needlework and quilting
- Writing short stories
- Storytelling
- Novels
- Films
- Painting
- Creating a mandala
- Visiting art galleries
- Listening to music
- Dance

(From Johnson and Jackson,[2] Jackson and Sullivan,[3] Marshall,[4] Tapajos,[5] Peterson and Williams[6] and Williams.[7])

I would add that a mind map, on which the individual can use words or pictures, could also be included in the above list.

It can be seen that some of these creative activities are 'active' – for example, where the students produce a piece of artwork, a video or some creative writing – while others are 'passive' – for example, where the students engage with art using the senses (i.e. sight, hearing, touch, taste and/or smell).

The use of the creative arts may well be dependent on the resources that are available in the learning environment. Creative writing is an inexpensive activity, as is the utilisation of poetry or novels for discussion purposes, and these aspects have been explored in Chapter 7. Art materials such as pens, paper, paints, scissors and glue are reasonably inexpensive, and the teacher may accumulate an increasing amount of resources if they use this strategy frequently. A colleague of mine who often uses this teaching strategy keeps a large carrier bag in her office that is full of old magazines and journals for cutting up to make collages and posters. Similarly, I maintain a small box of art materials and also have a box of building bricks which I use when covering research topics.

Materials for needlework and quilting can be more costly than paint and paper, but again if the teacher uses them often, the chances are that they will quickly accumulate. Having textures for students to work with provides a tactile experience and can help them to associate concepts such as pain. For example, wool may be itchy, sacking may feel rough and abrasive, starched cotton may feel stiff and uncomfortable.

Creative arts such as photography and video recording require more equipment, some of which can be expensive. It is possible that your local learning resources centre or library has a loaning scheme that would enable you to access these resources. Utilisation of these facilities may require additional learning (e.g. learning how to use a digital camera and edit the results), so incorporating them in a teaching strategy will require forethought. A discussion of the use of these media as a teaching strategy would require a chapter in its own right, and therefore the following account focuses predominantly on the use of art.

When using this approach it is important to consider the learning style of the individual student,[8] and one should bear in mind that the use of active strategies will possibly suit the activists and pragmatists, whereas the theorists and reflectors may prefer a passive strategy. Similarly, if you want the student to produce a creative piece then you may also need to consider the multiple intelligences involved[9] (*see* Chapter 1), such as bodily kinaesthetic intelligence or spatial intelligence, which may either enhance or hinder the student's *perceived* ability to create. Note that I have emphasised the perceived aspect of creativity, as a student may comment 'I can't draw' when in reality they can. What they might possibly be expressing at this moment is a fear of being judged by their efforts. It is incumbent on the facilitator (and I use that word pointedly, rather than 'teacher', as you are not there to teach them art) to promote a safe environment to allow the reticent student time and space to explore the materials and concepts under discussion.

In addition to the above, the concept of neurolinguistic programming (NLP) considers that individuals use a preferred mode of thinking – in sounds, pictures and feeling.[10] So while one student might enjoy music, another might prefer using paints to produce some artwork, and yet another might prefer a tactile experience such as using clay or different fabrics.

Advantages of using creative arts

One of the immediate advantages of the use of creative arts in healthcare education is that it differs from traditional lectures. This raises the interest and impact value for the student. The use of creative arts as a teaching strategy is often considered to be fun and recreational, and may therefore be effective in reducing daily stress.[6] However, its use goes deeper than just a 'fun' exercise, for it can help in all of the learning domains.

In the first, or cognitive, domain the use of creative arts can encourage non-scientific thinking such as metaphor-based thought, meditation and discussion.[5] One example, given by Cruickshank,[11] cites a discussion of artwork produced by a group of students, where the drawing of lips persistently represented the concept of communication, rather than using listening ears. The lecturer was able to highlight what was missing as well as identifying what was present. Similarly, perceptions can be explored. For example, when considering the question 'What do we mean by old age?',[12] each student drew their own image as they imagined themselves at the age of 75. The results showed a negative view of their future, with disability and death being prevalent. Both of these examples help to illustrate 'where the student is at' compared with where they might be, which is where the discussion aspect takes over.

It has also been suggested that the use of creative arts can increase intellectual and sensual aesthetic reactions[5] and critical awareness,[1] and can help to foster observational, analytical and interpretive skills.[5] It can aid the exploration of abstract concepts such as caring, suffering and pain,[3] which are so fundamental to the healthcare professions. Similarly, the cultural use of art and symbols can be examined.[3] If students have been asked to produce artwork at different stages of their course, then comparisons can be made between 'before' and 'after' pictures,[4] helping to demonstrate the student's cognitive development and thought processes – that is, whether 'where the student is at' has changed at all.

I can recall working with a student who had reached the end of her student nurse education and was making up time following sickness. We were both working in orthopaedic outpatients, and I was assigned as her mentor. At our first discussion I asked her to make a mind map of her orthopaedic knowledge. After she had completed the task I noted that there was a lot of empty space, and this helped us to formulate her learning plan. At the end of her placement we repeated the exercise, and this time the page was almost completely filled. This example demonstrates that the use of creative art could also be utilised as an assessment tool.

Another advantage of using creative art as a teaching strategy is that it helps to address the second domain (the affective domain) because it encourages reflection.[5,11,13] Producing a reflective drawing enables the student who does not often voice an opinion, or who tends to defer to more extrovert group members, to have an arena where they can express themselves.[11] What students draw can display rich and meaningful experiences[11] – a sentiment shared by one of my colleagues who used students' artwork as part of her Masters degree research into dyslexia, and found that she had an abundance of material to analyse. The use of artwork can impart awareness of personal values and feelings,[5] so students can express their positive and negative reactions to a piece of art, a photograph or a video and explore why they might feel that way. This emotional response can help to identify the degree of empathy experienced by the student.

It has also been suggested that producing artwork aids the development of intellectual and psychomotor skills, such as spatial vision and the ability to think in three dimensions[5] – a useful attribute if you are performing an operation or similar clinical task – and therefore addresses the third learning domain, namely that of psychomotor skills. I have certainly met a few surgeons who have produced works of art as a hobby, so perhaps the two are interlinked, with a need for a steady hand for both jobs!

If producing artwork is a group activity, as for example in the joint production of a mandala,[4] then the group dynamics can be observed by the facilitator, and this opens up a discussion of the concept of teamwork. Again, as the facilitator it is important to note that you are not just presenting the students with the activity, but also their artwork will then become the platform for a discussion.

However, if you are delivering a lecture then it is possible to let the students take a passive role, and you can put on a display of artwork. This is a fairly simple process if you are using a software package such as PowerPoint, as pictures can be downloaded from the Internet. In this way slide shows can be stored and easily changed depending on the topic currently under discussion. However, it can be expensive if you are using overhead-projector films (although these can be made into slides for use in a slide projector), although this is rapidly becoming outmoded twentieth-century technology.

Disadvantages of using creative art

One of the most obvious disadvantages of using creative art is that it may not suit large groups,[14] so consideration should be given to reducing the group size if active participation is required. In addition, one must bear in mind the students' reaction to this teaching strategy, which may be dependent on their previous exposure to use of this medium.[14] Conversely, if this is the first time that they have encountered creative art, it may take time for the students to become familiar with the medium.[14] Therefore it is important not to be downhearted if your initial flirtation with the strategy doesn't appear to work. Perseverance is the key – that and the enthusiasm of the tutor.[14] It has been pointed out that lecturers who have adopted this learning strategy have sometimes been considered 'eccentric' by their colleagues.[14] However, all fledgling strategies have had this response before being adopted into the mainstream system.

Before you embark on the use of creative arts, it is important to consider whether a supportive environment exists.[11] Students will not want their drawing ability to be ridiculed by the lecturer or their fellow students. Even a passive session, such as watching a video, might require cognitive preparation to be given to allow for emotional responses, together with time for a debriefing.

CASE STUDY 9.1

I was showing a first viewing of a video to a group of students. The video showed healthcare professionals talking about their experiences of dealing with death and dying. The last vignette on the video featured a staff nurse working in an Accident and Emergency department, who dealt with a mother and child who had been involved in a road traffic accident. The staff nurse suddenly stated that the child had been decapitated in the accident. I heard a chorus of horrified gasps emanating from the students, and I realised that I had not adequately prepared them.

When I was working with subsequent groups I informed them of the content of the video, and made particular reference to the details that they would hear from the staff nurse, before showing them the video. I elaborated on the details in a stepwise fashion:

1. male staff nurse talks about dealing with death
2. death concerns a child
3. the child sustained '*horrible injuries*' – the actual words used by the staff nurse, to serve as a cue when watching the video
4. the 'horrible injuries' referred to involved decapitation.

This cognitive preparation certainly reduced the shock impact on the students. I also ensured that adequate time was given for discussion of the contents of the video, which helped when debriefing the students.

A decision might have to be made as to whether it is a creative self-expression session or a discipline-based art education programme. If it is the latter, the lecturer may need a background philosophy of art education, with accompanying art-critiquing skills.[5] However, even if he or she does not have these specific skills, a lecturer should consider the appropriateness of the art chosen.[13] Students may need the link between the medium and their profession to be made clear to them.[14] This is especially true for healthcare professionals, who are so used to using a scientific mode of thinking.

If the session is an active, self-expressive session, consideration must be given to the available resources, to ensure that there is sufficient paper, paint, pens, pencils, etc. for all of the students. As the creative process cannot be hurried, it should be noted that it could be time consuming. This aspect can be dealt with effectively by giving the students a set time frame (e.g. an hour in which to produce a set piece). Once the students have produced their artwork, it may need 'verbal interpretation to clarify meaning and mutual understanding.'[11] This requires a dialogue between the artist and the audience, and if the group size is in double figures, again this can be a time-consuming process. It has been suggested that drawing may only represent espoused theory, not practice,[11] so it is important not to read too much into creative works, which are just that – creations.

Finally, creativity is a right-brained activity,[15] and therefore may not suit the student's preferred mode of thinking. I can recall an instance when I gave each student in a group a blank sheet of A4 paper and asked them to draw 'what it means to be a nurse.' The group was predominantly female, and the only male in the group had a frozen look on his face as he looked at the paper. I asked him what was troubling him and he explained that he 'couldn't think of anything' and that he couldn't do the exercise. When I asked if it would be easier for him to write down words, he readily drew up a list. On the basis of this I concluded that he might have been a left-brained thinker.

Summary

The use of art and the humanities is not often taught to healthcare education teachers, and it has been left to those who have actually experienced it as a student to develop it as a teaching strategy. It has been demonstrated to be a useful teaching strategy that can address all three domains if the activity is active, but which will also meet the cognitive and affective domains if the activity is passive. The emphasis in this chapter has been on the use of art, but the use of video media has also been mentioned.

It is clear from Box 9.1 that there are many creative activities that could be adopted for use in healthcare. For example, the use of video recording as a means of assessing communication skills is coming to the fore. Narrative writing is another creative activity that is receiving a lot of attention. Field trips to an art gallery have been used within my teaching establishment, and the students valued the experience and the change of environment.

It has also been noted that using the creative arts involves a resource cost in terms of facilities and equipment. These can be humble, such as pens and paper, or sophisticated, requiring additional skills, such as the use of a digital camera or video recording. However, the rewards in terms of learning and engagement with the topic need to be weighed against the financial outlay.

- ❑ Creative activities are perceived as being fun.
- ❑ They can be used for all three domains of learning.
- ❑ Students can be active or passive, depending on the activity.
- ❑ Creative activities enhance reflection.
- ❑ They may not be suitable if student numbers are high.
- ❑ Previous exposure to creative activity may enhance or detract from learning.

References

1　Hansen DT. A poetics of teaching. *Educ Theory.* 2004; **54**: 119–42.

2　Johnson A, Jackson D. Using the arts and humanities to support learning about loss, suffering and death. *Int J Palliat Nurs.* 2005; **11**: 438–43.

3　Jackson D, Sullivan JR. Integrating the creative arts into a midwifery curriculum: a teaching innovation. *Nurs Educ Today.* 1999; **19**: 527–32.

4　Marshall MC. Creative learning: the mandala as teaching exercise. *J Nurs Educ.* **42**: 517–19.

5　Tapajos R. HIV/AIDS in the visual arts: applying discipline-based art education (DBAE) to medical humanities. *Med Educ.* 2003; **37**: 563–70.

6　Peterson TO, Williams JK. So what does dance have to do with it? Using dance to teach students about leadership. *Decision Sci J Innov Educ.* 2004; **2**: 193–201.

7 Williams B. Collage work as a medium for guided reflection in the clinical supervision relationship. *Nurs Educ Today.* 2000; **20:** 273–8.

8 Reece I, Walker S. *Teaching, Training and Learning: a practical guide incorporating FENTO standards.* 5th ed. Sunderland: Business Education Publishers Ltd.; 2003.

9 Gardner H. *Frames of Mind: the theory of multiple intelligences.* London: Fontana; 1993.

10 O'Connor J, Seymour J. *Introducing Neuro-Linguistic Programming: psychological skills for understanding and influencing people.* London: Thorsons; 1990.

11 Cruickshank D. The 'art' of reflection: using drawing to uncover knowledge development in student nurses. *Nurs Educ Today.* 1996; **16:** 127–30.

12 Roberts S, Hearn J, Holman C. Using drawing to explore student nurses' perceptions of older age. *Nurs Older People.* 2003; **15:** 14–18.

13 Hodges HF, Keeley AC, Grier EC. Masterworks of art and chronic illness experiences. *J Adv Nurs.* 2001; **36:** 389–98.

14 Grindle NC, Dallat J. Northern Ireland – state of the arts? An evaluation of the use of the arts in teaching caring. *Nurs Educ Today.* 2001; **21:** 189–96.

15 Edwards B. *Drawing on the Right Side of the Brain.* London: HarperCollins; 1993.

CHAPTER 10

Simulation: transforming technology into teaching

Steve Hardman

Introduction

The use of simulation as a teaching strategy within healthcare education has taken off in the last five years. Simulation training has become a very fashionable accessory at most modern higher education institutes (HEIs) and healthcare trusts that are involved in healthcare education provision. Improvements in new technology and a decrease in the cost of simulation equipment have led to a substantial increase in the accessibility, availability and utilisation of simulation within a wider range of healthcare professional courses and curricula. Many HEIs and trusts are now investing substantial amounts of financial resources and teaching resources to provide simulation training for staff, but is it worth all the fuss? Is simulation a viable teaching method or just the latest fad in the provision of healthcare education?

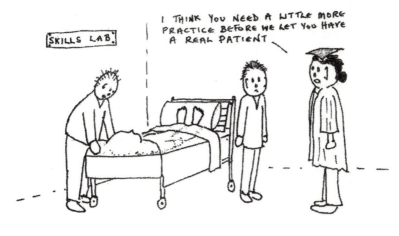

Within this chapter, it is my intention to try to answer these questions and, by referring to my own interest and experience in the use of simulation training, to discuss those topics that may lend themselves more readily to simulation. Key components, advantages, disadvantages and limitations of simulation training will be explored. It must be acknowledged at this point that the remit of this chapter is to provide an introduction to and brief overview of the topic of simulation, and that the discussion presented here is by no means exhaustive.

Reflection

Ever since I was a small boy, simulation has played an active part in my life. Having been awestruck watching *Star Wars* for the first in the Odeon cinema, I knew that it was my mission to train as a 'Jedi Knight' and to save the 'Rebel Alliance' from the evil 'Darth Vader' and the 'Empire.' Little did I realise that this required simulation equipment and training! My parents were tasked with providing the expensive simulation equipment necessary, namely a light sabre, batteries, regulation blaster, more batteries and authentic clothing! A suitably darkened room provided the ambience and realism of the 'Rebel Base' required for myself and several friends to begin the 'Jedi Knight' training programme that we had devised. Years on, it would appear that we may have been pioneers in the new simulation age!

Having moved on and entered the world of healthcare, during my training as a student nurse I found that simulation training again played its part in my development and the acquisition of much needed basic life support skills. These skills were honed upon rather unattractive and static resuscitation manikins. However, having survived the unattractive manikins, my future career path led me into critical care nursing and more contact with simulation training. This time, new skills of venepuncture and cannulation were taught on more realistic, but still low-fidelity, IV arms. It was not until I undertook a course in advanced life support that I came into contact with much more realistic simulation equipment and scenarios.

These were designed and set up to mimic the ward environment, which contained a seriously ill patient played by a moderate-fidelity simulator, and the hustle, bustle and stress of managing a cardiac arrest team, played by peers and faculty, correctly dealing with the dynamic situation as it unfolded and directing the team to treat the extremely unwell patient with appropriate interventions. This demonstrated clearly the possibilities of using simulation as an effective teaching strategy, using well-thought-out scenarios, realistic equipment and environments, with well-trained teaching staff and a thorough debriefing following the scenario.

My next major contact with simulation occurred when I entered the teaching profession, and a post teaching clinical skills to medical students. It was here that I first developed a true understanding of the importance, application and complexity of designing and undertaking simulation training as a teaching method. The role relied heavily upon the use of simulation, and was based on a well-thought-out curriculum design and a very well-resourced clinical skills department. Some of the simulation equipment that was used was of mind-blowing complexity, facilitating very detailed examination and reproducing minute detail. These simulators were high fidelity and very expensive to run and to maintain, but gave a very realistic representation of the clinical environment and clinical practice. Simulation was used successfully as an effective assessment method for the medical students, who undertook scenario-based objective structured clinical examinations (OSCEs) involving complex multi-station scenarios, simulation equipment, standardised patients and extremely good actors! I was now a convert to simulation training as an effective and exciting strategy for delivering elements of healthcare teaching.

If I needed any further evidence to convince me that simulation was an effective learning tool, this was provided by way of the British Army! Being involved with the Royal Army Medical Corps (RAMC) has provided invaluable experience of the almost limitless possibilities of using simulation on an extremely large scale! Of all the providers that are currently utilising simulation as a method of training, the military have truly embraced its full potential. Millions of pounds are spent on simulation training in the form of military exercises, scenarios are meticulously planned and resourced, and equipment is extremely realistic, as are the participants involved in the simulation. The aim is to simulate battle situations as realistically as possible, and from experience this is done extremely well, in the dead of night most often – and then whoosh! Trip flares, masses of concentrated machine gun fire (blanks of course), smoke grenades, flash bangs – it certainly makes your adrenaline flow. The British Army has also recently invested heavily in simulation equipment for training the multi-professional medical staff, purchasing many high-fidelity simulation models to use in military exercises. Again with experience of a simulated full-size military field hospital, amputee actors as simulated casualties, a great deal of make-up and fake blood, hectic triage areas, constant casualty drops, major incidents and enemy attacks, it is a sight to behold! Just don't expect to get much sleep!

Now I continue as an advocate of simulation, and am involved in teaching advanced life support courses around the UK. In my current role, I continue to utilise simulation alongside other teaching methods within an HEI, on both pre-registration and post-registration courses. Current projects include the development of a Masters level Advanced Practice course that will rely heavily upon the use of simulation as one of the key teaching methods. I have also been involved in the design and setting up of new purpose-built skills laboratories, furnished with necessary (but expensive) simulation equipment to facilitate training within both pre-existing and newly developed curricula.

Definition

So what is simulation and why is it being used now within healthcare education? It has been widely acknowledged that there is currently a boom in the use of simulation technologies, and many explanations have been offered for this. Within the realms of preparation of healthcare providers, emphasis has been placed upon fitness for practice, providing practitioners with appropriate clinical knowledge, skills and experience together with effective problem-solving skills for practice, and simulation may offer a way of facilitating this.[1] It has also been recognised that there is a need to develop healthcare practitioners in a safe and cost-effective way, in an experiential environment that provides opportunities for the development of decision-making, critical thinking and communication skills.[2,3] Again simulation may offer a solution to this dilemma, allowing students to train within a dynamic and realistic environment, encountering situations that may well be serious or uncommon in clinical practice, without threats to patient safety.[4]

Some authors suggest that the current increase in the use of simulation may be due to lower equipment costs and a realisation that simulation training offers a valuable and viable educational tool for training healthcare professionals.[5] The increase in simulation training has also been attributed to other factors, including the need to supplement the limited number of clinical placements for trainee healthcare providers and the emphasis on evidence-based clinical practice.[5] There is limited but growing acceptance that simulation has a positive outcome in terms of the student's clinical practice capabilities.[2] However, rigorous scientific evidence to support this is still limited at present.

The educational basis of simulation is the notion of experience. Students often state that they learn more when they have 'hands-on' learning and experience of situations. When students are questioned about this, they often claim that skills and knowledge make more sense and are easier to apply when working within the clinical setting. As stated previously, one of the aims of healthcare education is to equip students with and enhance the application of knowledge and problem-solving abilities within clinical practice. The fact that many students find these aspects easier, especially when undertaking 'hands-on practice', suggests that they could be experiential learners.[6] Experiential learning is an extremely important part of most healthcare programmes, as students undertake significant periods of time on 'practice placements', undergoing experiential learning within the clinical environment, and gaining valuable experience of their expected clinical roles.

The student's participation in clinical hands-on learning is expected to help them to understand and apply the cognitive and psychomotor skills that they have learned within the educational course, and to master the techniques and elements of problem solving that are relied upon by professionals working within clinical practice.[2] Simulation can provide significant experiential learning, but the environment and atmosphere that are created are extremely important, and have to be equivalent to reality to help suspend any disbelief and allow students to function as themselves.[7]

However, it would seem that the apparent recent uptake and explosion of the use of simulation within healthcare is somewhat misleading. Simulation training is not new, and there is evidence to suggest that it has been used in the healthcare setting for more than 15 years.[8–10]

To define simulation, it can be seen as the reproduction of the essential features of a real-life situation.[3] The aim of simulation is therefore to represent reality as closely as possible so that the student is convinced that the encounter resembles what would happen in a real-life encounter or situation.[5] This can be very difficult to achieve, and requires careful planning and facilitation of both the physical environment and the scenario that is used. It also requires the use of simulation equipment that is designed to replicate and resemble real-life patients, procedures or practice.

There are of course, different approaches to simulation, and various levels and types of simulation and equipment that are used. There are three main categories of simulation, namely computer-based simulation, task- and skills-based simulation and full-scale simulation. It is beyond the scope of this chapter to discuss the different categories of simulation in any great depth. However, the notion of fidelity of simulation will be discussed, and a brief overview of each category of simulation will be presented.

What is meant by the term 'fidelity'? The word 'fidelity' is often used within simulation to describe the level of accuracy presented or the precision with which the simulators or systems that are used actually reproduce reality.[3,5] As discussed previously, the aim of simulation is to produce an accurate representation of reality, so that the student is convinced that the encounter resembles what would happen in a real-life encounter or situation. In general, fidelity is often subdivided into three categories, namely low-, moderate- or high-fidelity simulation. These categories are relatively loose terms, and modern simulators can often be used as low-, moderate- or high-fidelity units.

- *Low-fidelity simulators* are often used as an introduction, allowing students to practise and acquire a new psychomotor skill. These simulators are static and are used to practise a single skill – for example, basic life support, venepuncture or injection techniques. They are designed to try to reflect certain anatomical structures or landmarks for practising the skill. They do not give an accurate or true representation of the real-life situation, but they do facilitate acquisition of the skill without risk to the patient.

- *Moderate-fidelity simulators* are a step up from the low-fidelity models, offering more realistic looks, design and features. These simulators tend to be useful for developing a deeper understanding of key principles and knowledge, allowing more thorough assessment to be carried out on the simulator. The manikins generally incorporate blood pressure monitoring, pulse monitoring, breath sounds, heart sounds and bowel sounds, together with correct surface anatomy and landmarks, and interchangeable limb and abdominal modules, to add flexibility and scope to scenarios. However, they often lack the accompanying physical movements, such as chest or eye movement. Many moderate-fidelity simulators can be programmed with basic computerised scenarios, allowing students to assess and detect certain dynamic changes. These units can also be used as a low-fidelity simulator for introductory training and skill acquisition.

- *High-fidelity simulators* offer the most realism by including realistic looks, sounds, movements, interactions and dynamic changes related to treatment. High-fidelity simulators are designed to allow interaction between the simulator and the student, often on both a physical and a verbal basis. This level of interaction can immerse the student in the simulation, facilitating a realistic experience. High-fidelity simulators are designed to accurately reflect the physiological changes that are seen with different conditions, in different situations and with physical and pharmacological treatments that are used. This level of technological realism facilitates the use of much more in-depth programmable scenarios, allowing students to practise complex psychomotor and assessment skills as well as to develop and hone key problem-solving and critical thinking skills within a safe and controlled environment. The high-fidelity simulators even provide feedback on the performance of the student in the use of interventions, so that management of the situation or condition can be accurately appraised.

Having considered the notion and levels of fidelity, I shall now give a brief overview of the three main categories of simulation, namely computer-based simulation, task- and skills-based simulation and full-scale simulation.

- *Computer-based simulation* relies upon software to replicate the situation or the subject being learned, and includes aspects of learning related to physiology, skills acquisition and critical thinking.[5] Computer-based simulation has the advantage that it may be available to students outside the normal hours of the university via Internet-based programmes. This may offer accessibility and convenience for many students alongside the promotion of independent learning, a key skill much sought after by many, especially HEIs and healthcare professions. The recent introduction of 'real-time' computer-based simulation gives an added element of fidelity to the programme. Computer-based simulation is tipped to become the dominant form of simulation used, as it not only offers convenience and accessibility, but also provides sought-after flexibility in relation to normal time constraints, content covered, assessment, analysis of the student's performance and debriefing.[5]

- *Task- and skills-based simulators* are the most widely used simulation systems at present. They facilitate the acquisition and honing of specific psychomotor skills and the development of sequenced tasks – for example, insertion of IV catheters. Often task- and skills-based simulators are low fidelity. However, newer moderate- and high-fidelity simulators are being introduced which include the use of virtual-reality technology and sensitive tactile feedback systems or haptics. As the student progresses in their learning of the skill, the fidelity of the simulator used can be increased to supplement their experience and learning, allowing fine-tuning of the skill for use in the practice setting. However, evidence supporting the application of skills-based simulation to practice is still scarce.[11]

- *Full-scale simulation* is an attempt to replicate the entire situation that is perceived by the student.[12] It involves the use of a high-fidelity simulator that is highly responsive and dynamic, so can reflect the actions of the student. The environment is also important, and is designed to resemble the real-life environment as closely as possible. Often this will include full-scale simulated units or ward areas, medical devices and equipment and consumables, as well as standardised patients, actors and role play. The whole intention is to envelop the student in the simulation, to convince them that it is 'real' and to facilitate crucial development of critical thinking, problem-solving, prioritisation and decision-making skills along with the use of appropriate psychomotor skills. On completion of the simulation, debriefing is used to share the common learning experiences and to revisit the learning outcomes of the session. Full-scale simulation requires a great deal of thought and planning, considerable physical resources and well-trained faculty to facilitate the simulation.

Advantages of simulation

Using simulation as a teaching method has definite advantages in healthcare education. The first and most obvious advantage is patient safety.[4,11] Simulation can provide a realistic and safe environment in which the student can gain and practise important evidence-based clinical skills.[2] Safety has become a high priority in clinical practice, and using simulation to master complex invasive skills and techniques is a quicker and safer way of learning.[13] As simulation training can be repeated many times, both the learner and the instructors are afforded a measure of reassurance, as mistakes cause no harm to the patient and the methods can be re-practised until the necessary skills have been acquired.[13]

Therefore a second advantage of using simulation is the fact that simulations can be reproduced time and time again and the student has repeated opportunities to practise their clinical skills and scenario management. Medley and Horne[3] have suggested that nursing students are constrained within their current clinical practice placements due to limited time, limited clinical resources, shortened length of patient stay and high patient acuity. Despite these constraints, students are still expected to demonstrate sound, safe clinical decision making, and this situation may well be generalised to all trainee healthcare professionals. Simulation technology may hold the key to overcoming these constraints, as the same clinical objectives could well be met through various simulated scenarios, in a safe, controlled and interactive environment that affords all students an equitable assessment opportunity.[3]

A third advantage of simulation training is the ability to replicate rare, life-threatening or complex clinical scenarios. Gaba[14] suggests that the most significant advantage of undertaking simulation training is the opportunity to present crisis-management scenarios without risk to the patient, and these scenarios can be repeated until proficiency in the recognition and management of these situations is developed. This use of simulation is further supported by Chopra *et al.*,[15] who suggest that exposure to these rare, life-threatening events helps the student to develop the ability to take appropriate action to avoid disaster. Simulation has been used for many years in the field of advanced life support, but has more recently been incorporated into many more scenario-based short courses within the healthcare setting, including the immediate life support and ALERT courses. Both are used effectively to educate multi-professional healthcare staff in the recognition and treatment of relatively uncommon but life-threatening events.

Alongside the advantages described above, several other benefits of using simulation have been suggested. These include the ability to create a dynamic and unfolding set of events that display the consequences of interventions used, and the opportunity to achieve increased fluency of performance in multifaceted tasks.[16]

This is further supported by other studies which suggest that simulation enhances cognitive, psychomotor and communication skills in students.[2,4,15] In addition, it is recognised that other professions have used simulation training successfully for many years in order to develop cognitive and psychomotor skills and performance in both commonplace and adverse-event scenarios, in particular the aviation industry, which invests many millions of pounds in a single flight simulator to train jet-aircraft pilots.[13]

Simulation as an educational tool makes inherent sense, providing much needed hands-on learning and experience for the student.[5] Further advantages include the fact that errors can be addressed during the simulation, and feedback from peers and faculty can be given immediately. This helps to prevent the student from developing poor practice by repeating the error over and over again without correction, and it also gives learners an appreciation of the problem as viewed through the eyes of others.[17]

Medley and Horne[3] have suggested that communication, teamwork and delegation can be integrated within the simulation scenario, and a mix of both technical and non-technical experiences can be offered by simulation. Simulation training not only increases achievement but also increases student confidence,[2] active participation, active learning and consistent and comparable experiences for all students who are undertaking the same simulation programme or scenario.[4]

Disadvantages of simulation

Having briefly acknowledged some of the key advantages of using simulation, I shall now consider the major disadvantages. From experience, the main disadvantage is the lack of planning involved before simulators are purchased and simulation is adopted as a blanket teaching method within an institution. It has been suggested that simulation training is typically adopted by institutions using a three-step approach:[5]

1 deciding that simulation is interesting
2 sampling the equipment available and purchasing simulators
3 gathering support for the use of the equipment and simulation within the programme.

It is often following on from the third step that problems occur, because little thought has been given to integration of simulation within the curriculum, or course infrastructure, who will teach it, and training of the faculty in the use of equipment or simulation as a teaching method.[5] Therefore it is important to realise that careful thought and planning with regard to the organisation, facilities, curricula, faculty and equipment are needed before jumping in with both feet and implementing simulation training.

Another key potential disadvantage of simulation training is the financial cost. Although the cost of simulation equipment has fallen in recent years with the advent of lower-cost alternative models boasting high specification and high fidelity, simulation remains an expensive business.[5] As well as the simulators themselves, which range in price from a few hundred pounds to around £30,000 for an average high-fidelity simulator, facilities to house the simulators are required. This often involves the design and construction of specific facilities, or the refitting of pre-existing premises, which may prove expensive.[5] Cost is also a factor in the provision of faculty to run the simulation training, and training of the faculty in the use of simulation equipment. The staff who will be using the simulation equipment will require training to become skilled in its use, to explore the full potential of the equipment and thereby facilitate and maximise the learning opportunity that it provides.[3]

Time could also be viewed as a potential disadvantage of setting up and using simulation. As with anything new, it may take time for other members of the teaching faculty to accept the introduction of simulation as a method of teaching within curricula. It is important that the trust of the staff is gained, that any questions about simulation training are answered fully, and that the limitations of simulation as a teaching method are acknowledged, along with its strengths.[5] As was mentioned earlier, the training of faculty is important but can often be time-consuming. The process of adapting a curriculum to support simulation teaching is an extensive and time-consuming one. The content that would be best taught through simulation needs to be determined, together with appropriate learning objectives for each simulation session.[3]

Meticulous design of the simulation scenarios is essential and requires careful consideration, as does the brief given to the participants involved in the simulation, including the students themselves. This, together with the physical set-up of the simulation to replicate reality, the facilitation of the simulation and the debriefing session to follow, is an extensive process and a time-consuming one. It is important that detail is included in the design and set-up of the simulation, even if it appears to be time-consuming, so that students become fully immersed in the scenario and thus gain maximum benefit from the learning experience.

Simulation topics

First, as a teaching method for healthcare professionals, simulation must not be viewed as a panacea. It has its limitations – not all of the topics that are taught on healthcare programmes lend themselves to simulation, and this must be acknowledged. Rystedt and Lindstrom[16] believe that simulation should be regarded as complementary to other forms of teaching and instruction, and I would certainly agree with this view. As for the topics that lend themselves to simulation, I am sure that a vast number are already used. However, the potential remains for many more to be developed.

From personal experience, simulation has been particularly useful in the teaching of fundamental assessment skills for pre-registration healthcare students, and leads on to the teaching of more complex assessment skills and the application of problem solving to both simple and complex clinical scenarios. This requires the use of a purpose-built simulation room – or 'skills lab', as most people refer to it – together with moderate-fidelity manikins and interchangeable modules.

Simulation has also proved to be an equally effective tool for teaching the assessment and application of management protocols for life-threatening situations, giving students the chance to practise the psychomotor skills involved as well as working through the decision-making processes and delegation issues that arise in these situations.

Rare clinical conditions and complications have also been simulated, along with sessions on the specific management of certain common clinical conditions that are seen on an everyday basis. I have found that one of the advantages of simulating common conditions is that it helps to overcome the complacency that can sometimes become apparent in some students, refocusing them on the need for thorough assessment and well thought out evidence-based interventions.

I have also been involved in a variety of simulations designed specifically as OSCE assessment tools, aimed at testing individual complex clinical skills, psychomotor ability and communication skills (verbal and non-verbal), as well as simulation OSCEs that assess combinations of decision-making, problem-solving, clinical and communication skills. Unfortunately, a discussion of the use of simulation and OSCE assessment tools is beyond the scope of this chapter. However, experience has shown them to be a useful combination that is worth exploring further.

There is still of course a great deal of further potential to be explored with regard to the application of simulation in healthcare education. With an understanding of the fidelity and the usefulness of simulation, as well as a recognition of its limitations, the number of topic areas and applications of simulation training will, I am sure, continue to grow and provide fascinating and stimulating educational and learning experiences for all involved.

Summary

Simulation and its use within healthcare education is not a new phenomenon, despite its recent increase in popularity and uptake as a teaching method. Simulation as an educational tool does seem to have become an accepted method of providing useful learning opportunities and experiences. However, it is acknowledged that there is a need for further evidence to support its use.

There are, of course, different forms of simulation technology available, including computer-based simulators, skills- and task-based simulators and full-scale simulators, each of which has different levels of fidelity in replicating the real-life situation. Fidelity is an important aspect to understand in relation to simulation, as it impacts directly upon what can be achieved when using simulation. All forms of simulation technology have their uses in teaching healthcare, and all of them also have their limitations with regard to what can be replicated and what can be taught.

There are definite advantages to using simulation as a teaching method within healthcare. These include maintaining patient safety, the ability to repeat situations, the ability to replicate rare and life-threatening events in a controlled and safe environment, and the dynamic and unfolding nature of simulation as an interactive teaching method.

It must also be recognised that there are certain possible disadvantages to using simulation, including a lack of preparation and poor integration within a course or curriculum, the expense of developing and using simulation within an institution (including financial cost), and the time-consuming nature of introducing, integrating and developing simulation training.

We are now working in exciting times. Simulation offers the potential for learning complex and dynamic elements of clinical practice in an interactive rather than static manner. Teachers need to familiarise themselves with the concept of simulation in order to understand the application and its limitations, and to fully exploit its potential. It must be remembered that simulation is not a panacea. It should be fully integrated into healthcare education in order to complement traditional methods of teaching and clinical practice experience, not replace them.

- ❑ Teaching staff require training in how to use simulation equipment.
- ❑ Simulation can be used to practise basic and high-level skills within a safe environment.
- ❑ Simulation enhances psychomotor and problem-solving skills.
- ❑ There are different levels of simulation equipment.
- ❑ Simulation equipment can be costly and may require a specific environment.
- ❑ Time is needed to write scenarios that make full use of the equipment's potential.

References

1 Roberts JD. Problem-solving skills of senior student nurses: an exploratory study using simulation. *Int J Nurs Studies.* 2000; **37:** 135–43.

2 Aliner G, Hunt B, Gordon R. Determining the value of simulation in nurse education: study design and initial results. *Nurs Educ Pract.* 2004; **4:** 200–7.

3 Medley CF, Horne C. Using simulation technology for undergraduate nurse education. *J Nurs Educ.* 2005; **44:** 31–4.

4 Fletcher JL. American Association of Nurse Anesthetists journal course: update for nurse anesthetists. Anesthesia simulation: a tool for learning and research. *AANA J.* 2005; **63:** 61–7.

5 Seropian MA, Brown K, Gavilanes JS *et al.* Simulation: not just a manikin. *J Nurs Educ.* 2004; **43:** 164–9.

6 Kolb D. *Experiential Learning: experience as the source of learning and development.* Englewood Cliffs, NJ: Prentice-Hall; 1984.

7 Streufert S, Satish U, Barach P. Improving medical care: the use of simulation technology. *Simulation Gaming.* 2001; **32:** 164–74.

8 Bond WF, Kostenbader M, McCarthy JF. Prehospital-based health care provider's experience with a human patient simulator. *Prehospital Emerg Care.* 2001; **5:** 284–7.

9 Freeman KM, Thompson SF, Allely EB *et al.* A virtual reality patient simulation system for teaching emergency response skills to US Navy medical providers. *Prehospital Disaster Med.* 2001; **16**: 3–8.

10 Gordon JA, Wilkerson WM, Shaffer DW *et al.* Practicing medicine without risk: students' and educators' response to high-fidelity patient simulation. *Acad Med.* 2001; **76**: 469–72.

11 Ziv A, Small SD, Wolpe PR. Patient safety and simulation-based medical education. *Med Teacher.* 2000; **22**: 489–95.

12 Seropian MA, Brown K, Gavilanes JS *et al.* An approach to simulation program development. *J Nurs Educ.* 2004; **43**: 170–74.

13 Haskvitz LM, Koop EC. Students struggling in clinical practice? A new role for the patient simulator. *J Nurs Ed.* 2004; **43**: 181–4.

14 Gaba DM. Improving anesthesiologists' performance by simulating reality. *J Anesthesiol.* 1992; **76**: 491–4.

15 Chopra V, Gesink BJ, De Jong J *et al.* Does training on an anaesthesia simulator lead to improvement in performance? *Br J Anaesth.* 1994; **73**: 293–7.

16 Rystedt H, Lindstrom B. Introducing simulation technologies in nurse education: a nursing practice perspective. *Nurs Educ Pract.* 2001; **1**: 134–41.

17 Goldenberg D, Andrusyszyn M, Iwasiw C. The effect of classroom simulation on nursing students' self-efficacy related to health teaching. *J Nurs Ed.* 2005; **44**: 310–14.

CHAPTER 11

Experiential learning exercises

Jan Woodhouse

Reflection

My earliest recollection of an experiential exercise as a teaching strategy takes me back to an English lesson in 1967. At the time the world was politically unstable, what with the Cold War raising the spectre of a nuclear attack at any time, and coverage of the Vietnam War being ever present in the press and news bulletins. For a teenager, as I was then, those were frightening times.

The English teacher arrived in the class and we waited to be set some work. However, he told us that there had been a news flash. China, he stated, had declared war on the USA, and we were to sit quietly because the bell was going to sound soon and we were all to go home. I sat there, thinking 'What's China got to do with

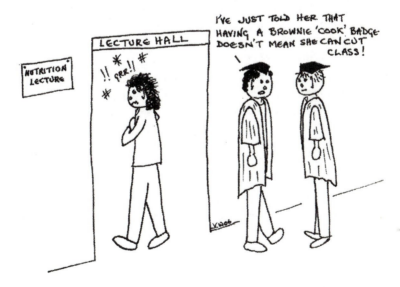

it?' I felt puzzled, asking myself 'Why haven't I heard about this before, and even if China has declared war on the USA – well, what's that got to do with us here in Britain?' The class sat in stunned silence as we waited for the bell to ring. Two, three, four minutes went by and then the English teacher stood up and said 'Take out your pens and notebooks and write about fear.' It was only then that the class realised that we had been had – that the 'news bulletin' was a lie and that we had been hoodwinked.

What my account shows is that the emotion that I experienced was not 'fear' as the English teacher suggested, but puzzlement. It also shows that as a result of experiencing that emotion I have remembered that session in the classroom, thereby demonstrating the power of an experiential learning exercise.

(As a postscript to my anecdote, a few years back I read of a similar story in a national newspaper. However, in that case the teacher was reprimanded for causing the schoolchildren unnecessary stress. This is a reminder that in today's classroom we have to act ethically and 'do no harm' to our students.)

Since then I have encountered experiential learning exercises in several different settings. One was on a management course. The participants were divided into several groups and given the task of producing greetings cards. Leaders were assigned to 'manage' each of the groups. However, the groups were unaware of the fact that each leader had been given a different style to act out – autocratic, democratic or laissez-faire. The groups responded accordingly, with productivity being highest in the democratic group, followed by the laissez-faire group, and the autocratic group downing tools and going on strike! There was a great deal of fun and laughter during this exercise.

Another encounter was during my Master's degree studies, although this time it was a lot more serious. The topic was 'personal process work.' A group of about fifteen of us were sitting in a circle, and we had just finished a discussion about our roles at work. The tutor started to question one of the students quite intensely. The student responded and the tutor probed further. The student continued to respond and the tutor continued to probe, to the point of bullying the student. This seemed to last a long time, although it was probably only a minute or so, but in that time the student had become flushed, was stumbling to find their words, and their body language was defensive. I felt uncomfortable witnessing this intimidating behaviour. I realised that if I spoke up I would risk being on the receiving end of the bullying, too, but I also realised that the heat needed to be taken off the unfortunate victim. I asked the tutor to stop his behaviour towards the victim. The tutor turned to face me 'You want me to stop?' 'Yes', I replied. 'Okay', said the tutor, and with that he moved on to a new topic.

Those of you who are familiar with the transactional analysis model of 'Victim, Persecutor, Rescuer' will recognise what happened in the above experiential exercise – the other student was in the role of Victim, the tutor was the Persecutor and I was acting as the Rescuer. This exercise helped me to gain an understanding of how I behave in groups and why I have sometimes had leadership thrust upon me. Through such experiential exercises I have undertaken interpersonal learning.

Definition

Rogers has commented that 'experience forms the basis of all learning', and from that learning comes the search for meaning.[1] So one might wonder why this book includes a chapter dedicated to the topic when it seems that everything we do could be classed as experiential learning. Sitting in the classroom is an experience. Working with patients involves gaining experience. However, the question one has to ask is 'Are we learning during the experience?' Ask a student what they learned during a particular placement and they may reply 'Nothing – I didn't gain anything from it.' This seems to indicate that there is more to experience and learning than first meets the eye.

Experiential learning has been defined as 'a sequence of events with one or more learning objectives, requiring active involvement by participants at one or more points in the sequence.'[2] Another definition is that it is learning 'that takes place as a result of an encounter with an experience that is planned by instructors within a course, programme (*sic*) or curriculum.'[3] The learning cycle of Kolb is often cited[1,4,5] in relation to experiential learning (i.e. the participant is exposed to a concrete experience, makes a reflective observation, processes the experience through abstract conceptualisation and will then move on to active experimentation). One important thing to remember here is that Kolb's model is circular, not sequential, and therefore the student may start at any of the four points.[4]

As healthcare education has a very practical basis, any time spent in the practice arena may well be regarded as experiential learning. But is that true for the classroom? Does sitting in a lecture count as experiential learning? My response to that question would be 'maybe', for my interpretation of an experiential learning exercise, when applied in the classroom, is slightly different to Kolb's cycle.

To support my interpretation, further writings make the point that experiential learning involves having hands-on activity,[6] facilitation and debriefing.[7,8] I propose that this is because, in the classroom, an experiential learning exercise *deliberately seeks an emotional response from the participant*. There is a concentration on the self, and participants are asked to speak in the first person[9] (i.e. use 'I' to denote that they own the emotional response). As one commentator puts it, 'it is the self interacting with the environment.'[10] Consequently, the definitive model I propose that best suits an experiential learning exercise in the classroom is that outlined in Box 11.1. Although some aspects of it can be applied to Kolb's model (e.g. the proposed activity equating with concrete experience), the proposed model acknowledges that the student may not always complete Kolb's cycle.

Completion of Kolb's cycle is dependent on the student's initial emotional response to the proposed task or activity. It is here that engagement with the topic, and subsequent motivation to take part, can be sustained or fail. Without engagement there can be no opportunity for the student to move on in the process of learning. There is then a second emotional response, which is to the undertaking and completion of the activity. The reflection on this stage now relies on the student and their level of emotional intelligence. Can they identify and verbalise the emotions that are felt? If they cannot, this may help to explain why one student may learn 'nothing' while another finds the experience meaningful and worthwhile.

The subsequent aspects of the stages are the verbalisation of the emotions felt, facilitated by gaining feedback from individuals. This may be achieved by giving each individual the opportunity to express what he or she felt. However, they should not be coerced into giving personal feedback, as they may not want to reveal their emotional responses.

During or after feedback, others in the group may want to share their emotions and reactions. On the other hand, the tutor and others may comment on what they observed and heard while the activity was being carried out or when feedback was being given. This usually generates a lot of discussion within the group. The final aspect of an experiential exercise is that of debriefing, which will be discussed later.

BOX 11.1 Stages of an experiential learning exercise

Proposed activity: problem solving, role play, artwork, game

First emotional response: to the proposed activity, which will lead to

Engagement or non-engagement: with regard to performing the activity. Students may be overt or covert about their level of participation

Second emotional response: to performing the activity

Reflection: on the emotional response to performing the activity

Feedback: from individuals on their (first and second) emotional responses to the facilitator and the group

Discussion: facilitated by the tutor and incorporating sharing and observations by other participants

Debriefing: by the facilitator, using a range of questions such as 'How do you feel?', 'What have we learned?', 'How can we apply what we have learned?' and 'Does anyone want a word with me in private?'

Advantages of experiential learning exercises

Experiential learning exercises can be used in any discipline. It can easily be seen both from my personal reflection and from the definitions that experiential learning in the classroom impacts on the affective domain. There are a variety of approaches that can be used as an experiential exercise, including role play, observation, listening to audio recordings/watching video recordings, research studies and simulation games.[8,11] Group work in which the participants are engaged in projects or reflection (such as clinical supervision) could also have an experiential element.[12] In addition, I would suggest that artwork and problem-solving exercises could be used as further strategies. The main point is that the student is involved with the activity or task. The experiential activity or task aims to build on previous knowledge, perception, cognition and experience.[5] Therefore it is an appropriate strategy to use with mature students, who represent a substantial proportion of students in healthcare education.

Experiential learning has been used to promote inter-professional learning,[3] a concept that is currently much promoted. It has been acknowledged that it enables community building, as well as raising of self-awareness.[5] This latter aspect is clear in my reflection, where I gained insight into how I react when I witness bullying. Self-awareness is the cornerstone of counselling education, and consequently the use of experiential learning is the predominant teaching strategy in this field. Counsellors need to know what might become a barrier to effective communication, so they reflect on their values, beliefs and attitudes. This prepares them for when they meet their clients in practice. Experiential learning, where it involves exposure to client groups, can reduce prejudice and combat discrimination.[13] Once again this emphasises the effect that experiential learning has on the affective domain. This is because experiential learning can be instrumental (i.e. bring about new knowledge) and supportive (i.e. provide the opportunity to discuss emotions).[5]

From an educative point of view, the link between acquiring knowledge and emotions is well recognised.[2,12,14] Experiential exercises have less structure to them, which allows for more meaningful acquisition of knowledge.[14] As you are building on previous knowledge and experience, you are able to transform these aspects of learning through intension and extension. Transforming through intension is achieved by the reflective element of the experiential exercise, and transforming through extension is the application of the new knowledge gained during the exercise.[5]

When these principles are applied to my memory of the management styles exercise, I can note that I had prior experience of the different styles of management, but until I did the exercise I did not have categories for them. During the exercise I experienced the autocratic style, and later learned about other categories (democratic and laissez-faire). I was able to reflect on my own style of management (transforming knowledge through intension), and when I returned to practice I was able to utilise the categories in particular situations (transforming knowledge through extension). For example, I may have acted as an autocratic leader in a cardiac arrest situation, rather than as a democratic one (who might lead a discussion on who was going to start cardiopulmonary resuscitation [CPR]!). In that practice situation, I would have been even less likely to have acted as a laissez-faire manager, leaving others to make up their own minds about whether to start CPR.

This illustrates the fact that experiential learning can bring about both 'formal learning' (course books, academia, meeting learning outcomes, testable), such as the categories of managers, and informal or 'unofficial learning' (observation, reflection, other books, untestable),[15] such as how management style is applied to personal practice. This means that, as a teacher, if you are using experiential learning exercises you must be prepared to expect the unexpected. The learning outcomes of the student may not match the intended learning outcomes of the teacher. However, these unanticipated outcomes may have a significant and positive impact on the student.[5]

Disadvantages of experiential learning exercises

It has already been stated that the participants need previous knowledge, perception, cognition and experience.[5] Consequently, it can be foreseen that if an experiential exercise is undertaken with students who do not have these attributes, it may come to grief, with the students muttering that they 'don't know what to do' or 'don't understand.' At this point they are expressing their first emotional response to the activity, and they may disengage and refuse (either overtly or covertly) to participate (*see* Box 11.1).

This would seem to indicate that you could not undertake an experiential exercise at first meeting. However, this is not the case. I recently attended an art therapy evening workshop, having not met either the tutor or any of the other participants before. During the introduction phase we were told that the evening would include an experiential exercise, so we had time to assimilate our first emotional response. In addition, the group all had counselling-type backgrounds and so, one could argue, were well used to the chosen teaching strategy.

The choice of activity may also be a disadvantage, and may well be dependent on the student's preferred learning style. I can recall participating in another experiential exercise in which there was a visualisation exercise followed by an art activity. We were required to draw the images that came out of the visualisation. One of the group members commented that she hadn't expected 'to be wasting her time drawing with crayons on a Masters course.' I would venture a guess that such an activity was outside her preferred learning style, whereas it suited mine perfectly.

However, as has already been noted, as a tutor or lecturer you cannot predict the emotional response to the exercise (remember the English teacher asking the class to write about 'fear' when I was feeling 'puzzlement'). It is important that the tutor pays heed to the process of an experiential exercise. For example, in my reflection on the Victim, Persecutor, Rescuer exercise, the tutor did not debrief us. The consequence was that some of the students, who had probably felt just as uncomfortable as I had (but did not speak out), thought that the 'persecution' exhibited by the tutor was a permanent aspect of his personality, and they withdrew from the module! One could also ask what happened to those who didn't speak out. Did they reflect and subsequently have a negative view of their capabilities when faced with a similar situation? This demonstrates that there could be a potential negative impact on the student. Therefore it is vital that all the stages of the exercise are followed.

Following the stages puts demands on the tutor and their teaching style, as it requires a facilitative approach. It also necessitates the ability to handle the whole range of emotions expressed by students, which can include anger, sadness, joy and grief, to name but a few. If negative emotions occur, the suggestions listed in Box 11.2 are aimed at providing a safe outlet for them.

I would also add that simply acknowledging the emotion might aid such expression. I frequently use an experiential exercise to help students to understand reactions to loss and grief. The emotions expressed are what I would call 'micro-emotions' – that is, they are verbalised emotions rather than ones which can be interpreted by a change in body language or behaviour. The range of emotions invoked has included anger, sadness, despair, concern, fearfulness and other similar negative feelings. On gaining feedback I simply record all of the students' responses on a whiteboard or flip chart, making no judgement about their responses. We can then discuss the similar emotional responses that they have witnessed with clients, patients or relatives.

BOX 11.2 Activities that allow expression of negative emotions

- *Mind-calming*: visualisation, relaxation.
- *Physical*: walking, exercise, stretching, game.
- *Dialogue*: talking with a partner, talking with a small group, sharing with the whole group.
- *Internal*: keeping a journal, self-assessment, goal setting.
- *Metaphorical*: put a rubbish bin near the door so that students can 'throw away' any negative feelings, either on paper or symbolically.

(From Jensen.[14])

It can be seen that this takes time, and that such discussions or other activities therefore need to be planned for. Similarly, the final stage of the experiential exercise – the debriefing – should also be factored in, otherwise the tutor's practice could be viewed as unethical in that it has 'done harm' (i.e. produced negative responses in the students). The Thiagarajan model of debriefing[8] uses the following questions to successfully debrief an experiential learning activity:

- 'How do you feel?'
- 'What happened?'
- 'What did you learn?'
- 'How does this relate to the real world?'
- 'What if . . .?'
- 'What next?'

Had this debrief occurred in the Victim, Persecutor, Rescuer exercise, I am certain that all of the participants would have returned to the module, for the safety of the learning environment would have been restored.

As with any activity where discussion takes place, it is often difficult to put a time limit on it. It is better to allow too much time for discussion than too little. I usually allow 20 minutes in my lesson plans, but sometimes the discussion will take longer, depending on the size of the group and the nature of the activity. However, sometimes the discussion and debriefing reach their natural end earlier than anticipated. So what should you do if the session finishes early? Well, students tend to like the odd five or ten minutes early finish, so you could say that you are giving back a positive emotion to them. Those few extra minutes may enable an individual who perhaps stayed quiet during the feedback to come and have a private word with you about their learning. It gives the tutor the chance to turn possible negative emotions into positive ones.

Having positive emotions builds trust and helps to create a safe learning environment – the type that actively encourages learning.[14] Using an experiential exercise requires a safe environment, and if the tutor does not have experience of providing such an environment, I would caution against using this teaching strategy. However, once confidence has been gained, the use of experiential exercises can be very rewarding for both student and tutor.

Summary

It has been shown that the term 'experiential learning' can be interpreted very broadly, in that some writers consider all learning to be experiential. However, another model has been offered with regard to experiential learning exercises in the classroom. In this setting, there is a sequence of stages that help to define an experiential exercise. This model helps to illustrate why some students learn through experience and others don't. Key aspects of an experiential exercise are activities designed to elicit an emotional response, facilitation of the process, reflection, discussion and debriefing.

The advantages of experiential learning are that it can be used with all professions and it enables learning in the affective domain. It particularly enhances the development of emotional intelligence, and for many individuals the session can be fun. However, the learning outcomes cannot be predicted, because the learning remains student-centred. This might be seen as a disadvantage.

Another disadvantage concerns the negative emotions that the student might experience. These can be offset by careful attention to all the feelings that are experienced and by a comprehensive debriefing. Time to allow for these processes should be factored into any session that uses experiential learning as a teaching strategy.

❑ Experiential learning strategies are especially useful for addressing the affective domain.
❑ Experiential learning exercises seek to deliberately invoke an emotional response in the student.
❑ Learning is student-centred, so learning outcomes are unpredictable.
❑ Positive and negative emotions may be elicited.
❑ Debriefing is an important element of experiential learning exercises.
❑ The learning that is gained can have a significant positive impact.

References

1 Rogers A. *Teaching Adults.* 2nd ed. Buckingham: Open University Press; 1996.

2 Walter GA, Marks SE. *Experiential Learning and Change: theory, design and practice.* New York: John Wiley & Sons; 1981.

3 D'Eon M. A blueprint for interprofessional learning. *J Interprofess Care.* 2005; **19:** 49–59.

4 Reece I, Walker S. *Teaching, Training and Learning: a practical guide incorporating FENTO standards.* 5th ed. Sunderland: Business Education Publishers Ltd; 2003.

5 Corbett AC. Experiential learning within the process of opportunity identification and exploitation. *Entrepreneurship Theory Pract.* 2005: **July issue:** 473–91.

6 Kwekkeboom KL, Vahl C, Eland J. Companionship and education: a nursing student experience in palliative care. *J Nurs Educ.* 2005; **44:** 169–76.

7 Brackenreg J. Experiential issues in reflection and debriefing: how nurse educators structure experiential activities. *Nurs Educ Pract.* 2004; **3:** 1–7.

8 Debriefing from www.thiagi.com (accessed 16 March 2006).

9 Owens PJ. Experiencing the other as the self: cultural diversity courses as liberating praxis. *Teach Theol Religion.* 2005; **8:** 245–52.

10 Baum N. Quality of life is not only for people served – it is also for staff: the multi-focal approach. *J Intellect Disabil Res.* 2005; **49:** 809–11.

11 Clark JM, Houston TK, Kolodner K *et al.* Teaching the teachers. *J Gen Intern Med.* 2004; **19:** 205–14.

12 Pololi LH, Frankel RM. Humanising medical education through faculty development: linking self-awareness and teaching skills. *Med Educ.* 2005; **39:** 154–62.

13 Coyle C, Saunderson W, Freeman R. Dental students, social policy students and learning disability: do differing attitudes exist? *Eur J Dent Educ.* 2004; **8:** 133–9.

14 Jensen E. *Brain-Based Learning.* Del Mar, CA: Turning Point Publications; 1996.

15 Chen W. Reading the word should be connected with reading the world: a lesson from Wordsworth and Hardy. *Educ Stud.* 2005; **31:** 95–101.

CHAPTER 12

Blended and e-learning

Debbie Robertson

Introduction

For some of us, the idea of 'e'-anything arouses feelings of fear and even dread. However, as we proceed in the twenty-first century, the Internet is now seen as an important part of modern life and, once we come to use and accept it, it offers us many sources of information and knowledge that can be accessed within a context of lifelong learning.

When we look at professional education, we can easily see how the use of Internet and computer-based learning has already crept into various aspects of course delivery, and the prospect and necessity of this increasing are acknowledged, albeit anecdotally, by many in the healthcare setting.

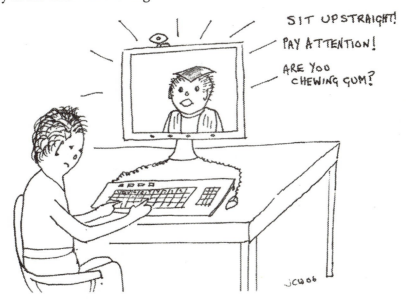

The subject of professional education has received a great deal of attention in the last few decades, with new and old strategies for teaching being compared and contrasted. Although some educators I have come across promote adherence to tried and tested methods of teaching, others tell me that using new and more radical strategies – both in the classroom and at a distance – can enhance the learning experience and promote more effective education.

It is generally accepted that each person attending a learning environment has individual needs and requirements according to their own learning style, which can influence how effectively they learn.[11] We must therefore look at how delivery of teaching materials by an e-learning or blended approach can be tailored to the learning needs of students. If students have different learning styles, then it must surely follow that educators have different teaching styles. This would be true whether the educator was delivering the learning materials face to face or using an Internet-based learning approach.

In this chapter we shall look at e-learning and blended learning strategies and consider how they may contribute to improved delivery of learning materials.

Definition

First let us look at e-learning and how it can be defined. It could be argued that if a person is learning in a way that uses information and communication technologies, then they can be said to be e-learning. This could be seen as a simplistic definition, but it does suggest to us that e-learning can mean different things to different people. For some it may involve use of Internet-based materials, while for others it may involve educational software or interactive programmes. The one constant in the definition of e-learning is the need for computer access. So given that context, what is blended learning? Blended or hybrid learning can be viewed as an integration of online or computer-based learning and more traditional forms of learning, such as classroom lectures.[2]

With the advent of the World Wide Web and the subsequent digital revolution, learning and information have become much more accessible to a wider range of people who wish to participate in learning but who have previously been restricted for many different reasons.

This has led to an explosion of individuals seeking e-learning or learning with a distance component. This has contributed to the idea that blended or hybrid learning is fast gaining pace as a more effective way to address learning needs in the twenty-first century.[3] However, blended learning is not without its critics, and has not been wholeheartedly embraced by all those in professional education,[4] as it can be seen to have as many disadvantages as it has advantages.

Education within the healthcare profession attracts learners from a variety of back-grounds, and sometimes the only common factor is that they are all adult learners.

Cross[5] suggests that, due to the different characteristics of the adult learner, programmes aimed at them should take into account several factors. She refers specifically to the need for choice in the 'availability and organization of learning programmes.' Adults entering the learning environment have different needs to school-age learners, and often have much to contribute to their own learning.[6]

What should we expect from an e-learning or blended learning approach?

I think that an effective e-learning package should aim to provide the right content at the right time for the student group at which it is aimed. It should be able to motivate students to learn and subsequently apply their knowledge and skills to practical situations. This can be achieved by providing learners with easy and immediate access to the content within an attractive and easy-to-use format.

Relating e-learning or blended learning to education

It seems that a common theme in adult education is a specific need with regard to the mode of delivery of information. In my experience, many adult students are returning to learning or are learning while continuing in full- or part-time employment, while some may have had to overcome significant barriers to their learning in order to enrol on courses. All of these needs must be addressed by the course design in order to enable all learners to be equally advantaged on their chosen programme of study. Therefore the category of adult learners provides a unique challenge in education, and the use of an e-learning or blended learning approach by the educator may facilitate learning in this group.

The educator has a multifaceted role in delivering information. They should be able to communicate the information effectively to the learner by whatever method has been chosen, and they should also be able to facilitate the learning occurring at that time. They play a huge part in motivating the learner, and it is therefore vital that they are highly motivated themselves. It is also important that they can reflect on their methods and modes of delivery and constantly evaluate the effectiveness of their education.[7] This reflection and evaluation should enable the educator to select methods of delivery of information that best suit their group of learners and, if they need to, consider a blended learning or e-learning approach.

Building a blended learning strategy

In order to build a blended learning strategy, the educator must select methods of delivery of learning materials that are relevant to the student group and the available facilities. Once an appropriate e-learning method has been selected, this can be hybridised with face-to-face contact sessions to form a true blended learning strategy.

The choice of how to deliver face-to-face contact sessions is varied and depends on many factors that are usually within the personal experience of the educator or their peers. These factors can include the size of the group to be taught, the resources available, the entry level of the learners and the expectations of all parties.

Recent opinion favours a move away from the didactic lecture format that was traditionally used to deliver information in a face-to-face session,[8] but this method of delivery should not be dismissed out of hand, as it provides an effective learning environment for many students, and can successfully be built into a blended learning approach.

How to make it work

Utilising the knowledge and experience of the adult learner to contribute to their learning experience may best be achieved by using different face-to-face teaching approaches. I think the use of group work and discussion forums can prove to be a good way of facilitating their learning. It also allows the educator to measure the learning that is occurring by observation and questioning during the face-to-face contact, something which I find is much more difficult to demonstrate using a pure didactic approach. But how can we do this effectively in a virtual learning environment such as online learning?

There are many ways in which students and educators can interact within an online arena. The availability of advanced software to allow synchronous online discussion and delivery of lectures to a virtual classroom is a prime example, but simpler and more widely used methods, such as asynchronous discussion boards and email, can be just as effective if used properly.

National opinion

Blended learning and the use of e-learning are advocated nationally by a number of professional and governing bodies as the way forward in adult education. Mary Wright[9] has outlined the need for flexibility in access to and delivery of learning materials within the context of continuing education for staff within the NHS. She also suggests that a common strategy should be developed in order to maximise effectiveness and minimise wastage of resources.

The national vision for e-learning in the NHS is to enable staff to access learning opportunities at times and places that best fit in with their lifestyle. This means 24-hour access to knowledge and learning resources, 365 days a year, from places that are most convenient for individuals and groups.[10] The Higher Education Funding Council for England (HEFCE) is 'committed to working with partners to fully embed e-learning in a sustainable way within the next 10 years.'[11] This statement suggests a high level of commitment to e-learning as part of a blended learning strategy in higher and health education for the future. This therefore puts a firm onus on us as educators to embrace blended learning and e-learning as an inevitable part of the future of healthcare education.

Advantages of blended learning and e-learning

From what we have seen above, one of the key advantages of a blended or e-learning strategy is the flexibility and accessibility that it offers and how this allows it to fit into modern society and its demands for education. It allows people to learn at their own pace with numerous opportunities to revisit and revise previous material as needed by the individual learner. It provides the motivated learner with seemingly limitless opportunity to enhance their learning experience at a time and place that is suitable and convenient to them.

This type of approach can also reach a much larger population of learners at one time than traditional teaching methods. Although it would be unwise to attempt to give a classroom lecture to 1000 students, this is not impossible or impractical using an e-learning approach. The online learning environment can also easily overcome boundaries of distance, with accessibility worldwide. The journey to college now becomes as simple as walking upstairs to your computer, attending a local college, library or Internet café to gain online access, or the ability to access coursework and materials from the workplace.

Another advantage of blended or e-learning is its suitability for multi-professional education. With this becoming a more common form of education in the arena of health and social care, this has the potential to make the adaptation of blended or e-learning to this form of education easier for the educator.

Disadvantages of blended learning and e-learning

There are a number of disadvantages to blended learning. The very components of blended learning that make it more flexible and accessible may in turn be some of the major barriers to delivery of the programme. Despite the fact that the technological and digital age is well and truly with us, a significant proportion of the population still do not have routine and consistent access to the Internet. This is exemplified by the fact that in the latter part of 2004 only 52% of households had online Internet access.[12] It could be said that by offering a blended learning approach we are advantaging the already advantaged and conversely disadvantaging the disadvantaged with regard to computer and Internet access.

Another technological problem is 'downtime.' This occurs when the server is unavailable for any reason, whether due to technical problems or routine maintenance, and it can lead to extreme frustration and anxiety on the part of the student. It is important to liaise closely with the computer services department within the institution to schedule routine maintenance at the least inconvenient time wherever possible. A good working relationship with the computer services department can make or break a blended learning or e-learning service.

Access may not be the only problem with regard to the technological side of blended learning. There are those who either do not or cannot avail themselves of the use of computers or the Internet. Computer literacy and ability are important prerequisites for any blended learning or e-learning programme, and this factor should be recognised before any learner enrols on a blended learning course.

With regard to other disadvantages, the aspect of personal motivation cannot be ignored. Attendance may be easily measurable in the classroom, but is much more difficult to measure with online learning or computer-based learning. The less motivated may not engage with the online materials in the most productive manner, and in a purely distance learning situation this could rapidly cause problems. Although this may not be so likely to occur with a blended approach, it may still be a cause for concern.

We should also consider attitudes towards computers and online learning *per se*. You may find that some students tend to have a very negative attitude to this type of learning, preferring face-to-face contact instead. This may derive, as I have found, from some of our students' only experience of learning, and it definitely relates back to their schooldays. As our generation progresses, and with computer-based and online learning now being an integral part of primary and secondary education, its incorporation into tertiary education may be less problematic.

Time considerations

The teaching of a blended learning or e-learning course can be extremely time consuming. Although much less time is spent in the classroom, this does not always mean that e-learning is time saving. In my experience, students often make greater use of email and discussion board facilities, which require monitoring and response by the lecturer. This can take up a great deal of time, especially if, as is often the case, student numbers on blended or e-learning courses are larger than those on classroom-taught groups. The use of group emails can save some time if several students are identifying similar problems.

Referencing e-material

Many of you will find that students on all types of courses, not just those with an e-learning component, are often using the Internet and online resources much more than before. This poses a potential problem for traditionally accepted forms of referencing style. The favoured Harvard and Vancouver styles provide little guidance on referencing e-material. Of the styles currently in use, the 'author-date' system from the American Psychological Association (APA) style offers most help with referencing e-material, and this may lead to it being adopted by many more institutions unless changes are made to other styles.

Application of a blended learning approach

In an attempt to understand why, when and how blended learning may be appropriate, we shall look at an example from my current teaching portfolio.

CASE STUDY 12.1

A blended learning approach has been applied to the Non-Medical Prescribing course. This course is open to suitably qualified nurses, midwives, pharmacists and other allied health professionals, namely physiotherapists and podiatrists. It will enable them to gain a nationally recognised qualification that allows them to prescribe medication under strict legislation and guidelines. It is run to meet the criteria set out by legislation and by the Nursing and Midwifery Council (NMC), the Royal Pharmaceutical Society of Great Britain (RPSGB) and the Health Profession Council (HPC).

The course comprises the following:

- 66 hours of direct contact, consisting of one full-day contact session every second week and two additional flexible contact sessions
- 80 hours of supported distance learning (SDL) using Web-based learning materials
- 90 hours (12 days) of supervised prescribing practice with an identified prescribing supervisor
- 216 notional hours of private/work-based study within specified directions of study.

The students who attend this course fall into a category of adult learners that provides us with a unique challenge in higher education. They are all in full- or part-time employment and are undertaking the course to enhance their job status and extend their roles as healthcare professionals to improve patient care and access to medication. Their employment status means that it is highly unlikely that they would be released from the workplace to complete a traditional full-attendance/full-time course. They come from a variety of different workplaces, backgrounds and geographical areas. They tend to be highly motivated, as this qualification can either be essential for their continuing employment or lead to an enhancement of salary. For these particular reasons it was decided that the use of a blended learning approach might be the best method of information delivery to facilitate learning in this group.

It can be seen from the above layout that the design of this course follows a true blended learning strategy and was devised in order to maximise recruitment to and retention on this course. As the students are in continuing employment while on the course, it was essential to design the delivery of course materials so as to ensure that it was possible for interested professionals to enrol and complete the course without detriment to either their employment or their learning.

Prospective students are informed of the course content prior to enrolment, and are therefore aware of the absolute need for good computer knowledge and skills and the ability to make use of the Internet and e-learning resources. The online learning section of the course website is divided into two main sections. The first section has online learning materials which the students can access and activities for them to work through in order to augment their learning and to help make the material provided more engaging. This section forms the e-learning part of the blended strategy. It is important that this area is a truly interactive learning environment and not simply an area of e-information. This is vital to ensure that the learners do not become bored by reading through page after page of content and therefore do not learn in an effective manner. As this course should be ever responsive to the needs of its students, a full evaluation of this e-learning area will reveal whether and how it has contributed to the learning process for the students, and therefore if it is as effective a teaching strategy as we perceive it to be.

The second section contains copies of the face-to-face sessions that have previously been delivered to the students. The purpose of this is to help the students to relate the information and activities with which they are interacting online to the learning that has taken place in the classroom. This integration of knowledge and information from both sources of delivery must take place if blended learning is to be effective. This duplication of information could be viewed by some as an inefficient use of resources. However, anecdotal evidence from current learners suggests that having the information from the face-to-face session available when they are accessing the online learning activities is more useful than not having it to hand, and actually facilitates their understanding of the e-learning materials. In future it will be worth formally reviewing this area with a view to assessing the effectiveness of duplicating this information. This represents an ongoing area of research.

Another valuable area of the website is the discussion board. This provides a useful forum for the students to interact with the tutors and the other learners in their cohort. It allows the free exchange of knowledge, information and opinion in a much less challenging environment than the classroom, and was welcomed by the students. It also acts as a lifeline between contact sessions, as they can use it to raise any problems with or concerns about any aspect of the course. However, the discussion board does seem to result in a plethora of complaints and banal and trivial comment, rather than a true e-resource to support learning. On reflection, this area of the website could be used to greater benefit with more direction being given by the educators and a more sound structure and format. This may best be undertaken by the setting up of threads at the commencement of the course, to direct the learners to areas which could appropriately be addressed by use of the discussion board, thereby hopefully avoiding its misuse.

One issue that was raised recently by the learners on the course at the University of Chester revealed a potential problem in delivering a course with a high proportion of e-learning. Some of the students were only being given study time by their employers to cover their face-to-face contact days. This meant that all online learning would have to be undertaken by the students in their own time, and this might be detrimental to their overall learning. Another issue that came to light was related to the issue of students undertaking the online learning in their own time. Many found it difficult to secure access to a computer and/or the Internet at home. This is an obvious barrier to their ability to work on the online course component, which might not have been a significant problem if their employers had given them the required study time so that the students could use that protected time at work or college or in the library to complete their learning objectives.

Conclusions

It seems clear that the development of teaching and learning strategies in higher education is a constantly evolving process and subject to many influences. Some strategies increase and decrease in popularity, often in a cyclical manner in response to the changing needs of learners, whereas the popularity of other strategies remains unchanged. With the advent of the Internet, and more and faster access to computers and all that this can offer, I think that the technological changes in the delivery of education will be a cornerstone for the development and improvement of lifelong learning strategies for the adult learner of today. The needs of the adult learner are differing and complex, and the factors that influence how, when and why they learn are equally diverse.

With the advocacy of many professional and governing bodies, demonstrated by their commitments and strategies with regard to this form of learning, it would seem that the place of e-learning in education is assured. As with any teaching and learning strategy, its success will be measured over time and its future will be decided on the basis of an evaluation of its effectiveness.

The use of a blended learning strategy would, on the face of things, effectively address the needs of the adult learner with regard to timing and delivery of course learning, materials and information, and utilising the flexibility of the online component of the learning programme. However, enthusiasm for this approach as the answer to how to teach adult learners should be tempered with caution. Barriers exist which can effectively prevent learners from accessing all areas of a blended learning course. Some of these barriers are well recognised and can often be catered for by setting requirements before the commencement of the course. Some other obstacles may not be easy to identify or to address, as they may be very individual, but may nevertheless prove to be a major problem for some learners.

For blended learning to be truly effective as a teaching strategy, it is important for the educators involved to recognise the strengths and weaknesses of this method, and to assess whether or not it is an applicable strategy for the particular course and student group that they wish to teach. If it fits the criteria for the course, and is set up and maintained appropriately, blended learning can prove to be an extremely effective way of delivering education to learners with complex needs.

- ❑ It provides a flexible approach to learning for many students.
- ❑ It provides a good medium for multiprofessional learning.
- ❑ It allows further education to be level and pace specific.
- ❑ Inadequate technical infrastructure and support can create a barrier to learning.
- ❑ E-learning materials must be designed to motivate and engage the student in the learning.

References

1 Honey P, Mumford A. *Honey and Mumford Learning Styles Questionnaire*; www.campaign-for-learning.org.uk (accessed 1 May 2005).

2 Thorne K. *Blended Learning: how to integrate online and traditional learning.* 1st ed. London: Kogan Page; 2002.

3 Kennedy DM. Standards for online teaching: lessons from the education, health and IT sectors. *Nurs Educ Today.* 2005; **25**: 23–30.

4 Oliver M, Trigwell K. Can 'blended learning' be redeemed? *E-Learning.* 2005; **2**: 17–26.

5 Cross KP. *Adults as Learners.* San Francisco, CA: Jossey-Bass; 1981; http://adulted.about.com (accessed 28 April 2005).

6 Forrest S. Learning and teaching: the reciprocal link. *J Contin Educ Nurs.* 2004; **35**: 74–9.

7 Cox P. *Online Learning: old wine, new bottles or a new way to learn in a post-modern society?*; www.nw99.net.au (accessed 9 May 2005).

8 Smedley JW. Working with blended learning. In: Hartley P, Woods A, Pill M, editors. *Enhancing Teaching in Higher Education.* London: Routledge; 2005.

9 Wright M. *The National E-Learning Strategy for the NHS*; www.nhsu.nhs.uk (accessed 9 May 2005).

10 Department of Health. *NHS Lifelong Learning Framework*; www.dh.gov.uk (accessed 9 May 2005).

11 Higher Education Funding Council for England. *HEFCE Strategy for E-Learning*; www.hefce.ac.uk (accessed 9 May 2005).

12 National Statistics Omnibus Survey. *Access to Internet from home – data from Family Expenditure Survey 2005*; www.statistics.gov.uk (accessed 9 May 2005).

CHAPTER 13

Self-directed study

Liz Sweet

Where to start: your actions

To start this chapter I would like you to reflect on the most recent assignment or lesson preparation that you have done. Where did you start when you were given a topic to teach or an assignment to write? Does your assignment develop in the same order as your study? Do you shuffle your notes and change their order from the order of your research findings? What happens at each rewrite? Does the order change yet again? These questions might imply that this chapter is about assignment writing or lesson preparation, but it is not. It is about self-directed study or the study route/ study journey that you take in order to produce a finished piece of work.

I started working on this chapter in a traditional way and tried an electronic

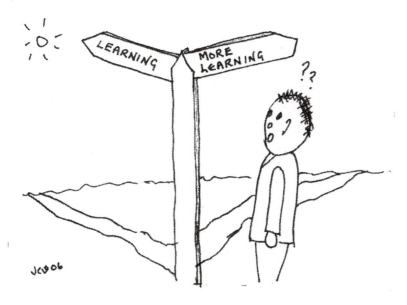

database search for 'self-directed study.' The findings were very limited. 'Study, self-directed' produced many references, but not 'self-directed study.' With each different database (Blackwell Synergy, Science Direct, Proquest) many references were found for 'self-directed learning' and its synonyms, but again not 'self-directed study.' This raised the question of why there were no direct references. What is it about 'self-directed study' as a single concept that means that the term is used frequently on timetables but not in the literature? The following chapter is my own 'self-directed study' journey as I explore my understanding of the term 'self-directed study.' The evidence is presented in an order that I hope is logical to the reader and the argument/discussion, but *not* necessarily in the order in which I researched the topic. The chapter is divided into three sections – the evidence or key viewpoints relating to the concept of 'self-directed study', a few exercises to help you explore your own self-directed study strategy, and finally a discussion of what this means for the role of the teacher/lecturer. The evidence of my reading and thinking has been divided into focused sections with a main theme. The themes become more complex, and each in itself is an area of significant debate.

Each selected theme has been scrutinised via literature review and analysis of experience. The literature review is based on over 30 years of reading nursing and education literature, so I have only identified the key texts which I now realise have shaped my thinking over the past years, as it would be impossible to reference all that I have read. The key elements selected are referenced by the reading that triggered my thinking, related to each theme. Against each theme is a number which identifies the order in which each concept is studied, showing how the order of study may either show or appear to have little relationship to the order of writing or use.

The real purpose of the chapter

My self-study journey is now documented. I have used the writing of this chapter to undertake an analysis of my own study journeys. It is hoped that this will illustrate how self-directed study is unique to each individual. Consequently, each person needs to become familiar with their own study routes, and facilitators of learning need to be able to foster this self-awareness by not always assuming that their way is the best.

Theme 1: module hours (concept 10 in my study order)

When you look at any handbook for a module, which is worth 150 hours of student effort, then for a level 2 module there will be 25 to 35 hours of contact time, and the rest is self-directed study. This amounts to over 100 hours! This is a lot of time, which can make or break a student's success with a module. For students of nursing, medicine or other practice-based courses there will also be an equivalent number of hours in practice. What do students do with this time study and practice? How do they structure it and what do they see as successful use of that time?[1,2] (*It was interesting to me that this theme only became overtly relevant when I started writing the chapter rather than researching it. I have been using the contact time and self-directed study formula for many years, and it is now assumed knowledge.*)

Theme 2: working to pass an assessment/meet targets (concept 7 in my study order)

It is commonly agreed in the educational literature that students study in order to pass exams rather than 'reading the subject.' Successful study for some students may simply mean success in assessment. Curriculum planners and module leaders frequently discuss this when reviewing assessment strategies and activities. When considering professional education, is it sufficient for students to be assessed in some elements of the module/programme, or should they demonstrate knowledge and competence in all elements of all modules? This is a debate that continues both in the Quality Assurance Agency (QAA) literature and between educators.[3]

Theme 3: whose theory? (concept 2 in my study order)

What is theory? In my view it is simply a mental extraction or juxtaposition of concepts which are put together to help the researcher and reader to understand the real world. It is the intellectual tool used to enable people to talk about the same things and explore the implications for the real world without too much misunderstanding. One theory does not fit all. An example here is learning theories, of which there are many. None of them fully explain learning, and new ones are generated each time additional information and tacit knowledge become explicit.

Theme 4: tacit knowledge (concept 1 in my study order)

Theory can only explain and communicate what is known or perceived. However, it is well recognised that activities in the workplace are influenced by 'theory in action' (i.e. that which is known but cannot be explained). This is further supported by research on clinical decision making and 'pattern recognition.' An experienced practitioner will make a correct judgement on the basis of apparently less information than a novice. The novice will need and be expected to work systematically through the full assessment, and may then make a judgement. Experts will explain what works in practice. This explanation may not always be congruent with espoused theory, thus setting up a conflict for the learner. Which is correct – written theory or what is observed and works in practice?[4]

This was the first area of consideration in my study journey because it is here that the question 'How does the topic relate to practice?' fits. It fits in, for me, by a brainstorm, which answers the question 'What do I see happening in practice related to, in this case, self-directed study?' If I were preparing a session on sociology or psychology and healthcare, I would be asking the questions 'How have I seen people behave in a healthcare context? What, in their pasts, and from my experience with other people, may influence that behaviour?' This is where I have had to learn that my initial assessment of a topic may not fit a logical, theoretical approach. But my experience tells me that it is the balance between the two that produces teaching which is alive and really relates the concepts of theory and practice for students.

Theme 5: electronic resources and cognitive overload (concept 4 in my study journey)

Over the past decade the availability of electronic resources for learners has expanded exponentially. This means that learners have no excuse for not accessing the literature, but it also means that they can get lost in it, be sidetracked or follow an inappropriate line of exploration (from the viewpoint of the module leader or marker of their work).[5] Using core texts appears to be a thing of the past, and reference to primary sources is now required, regardless of how long it takes the learner to access these and read the full text rather than another author's simplified explanation. I am not advocating academic anarchy, but consider the implications for the learner in perceived wasted time. Furthermore, why does the Open University supply the core reading for each module rather than encourage students to access *any* tangential literature? It could be argued as implicit in this that perhaps rather than quantifying modules in terms of student effort, scope of learning may be more appropriate. The QAA would argue that this is achieved by the way in which the learning outcomes of the module are written. I would dispute this, as many students only work to pass an assessment rather than to 'read' the subject,[4] but this debate is beyond the scope of this chapter.

A more serious issue related to the wide range of electronic resources available is the question of whether students use the academic logic on which the module outcomes are based to guide their study or their own developing tacit knowledge. When using tacit knowledge one must be prepared for a long learning journey before one can guarantee that all the accepted and expected academic reading has been covered.

As an experienced literature searcher, I can scan-read abstracts and assess their relevance to my current study topic, but the novice student may take longer and be taken down blind alleys. However, 'reading' a subject rather than target reading does eventually pay dividends.[6]

Theme 6: thinking time (concept 3 in my study journey)

What is thinking time? I am not sure, but from personal experience I know that I prefer time between reading a new topic for teaching and delivery of the session, to allow my brain to 'mature' my understanding of the work. For me the ideal is 8 to 10 weeks' notice of teaching a new topic. I read a range of material, surf abstracts for the general topic area in order to familiarise myself with key words, concepts and authors, and then undertake a more detailed literature search and reading. My target here is to produce a diagram or table that encapsulates the association of ideas and concepts as they apply to my understanding of practice. I then put the work away and 'forget' about it until 2 or 3 weeks before the teaching session, when I produce the lesson plan and materials. During the intervening time I find myself triggered into thinking about the new material by conversations, observed events and media sound bites. I find that these associations are essential if I am to be able to explain not just the theory studied, but its potential application to the real world. During this time I am testing the 'fit' of the new knowledge with the way I have seen the world, and as necessary I review the way in which I see the world. This is a painful process for some when they realise that their own way of viewing the world is limited, inappropriate, or misleading their judgements. When learning has not become a way of life, change is resisted rather than embraced.[7–9]

Theme 7: my personal view of learning (concept 9 in my study journey)

'Lifelong learning' is a term that is frequently bandied about. But what does it mean? This is not an exploration of the concept of lifelong learning, so I will just describe my own viewpoint here, and what it means to me. Recently a colleague was describing their experience in clinical practice. It was interesting, amusing and above all informative for its description and analysis of practice. However, my colleague made an interesting comment to me. They thought that I listened, took that new knowledge and would internalise it and use it in my teaching to help to explain a situation or theory to learners. My second-hand knowledge was becoming part of my learning to use in my work.[10]

This now brings me to a simple personal definition of 'self-directed study' as any activity that enables me to understand, and undertake in this case, my role as teacher. It can be any activity – for example, searching for information, reading, watching television, listening to others or just thinking. In other words, life is 'self-directed study', but the outcome of that study is given a different value depending on the context of its use (e.g. assessment results versus depth of understanding, custom and practice versus creative solutions to problems, successful anticipation of change agendas versus following the political policies and traditions of the area of work).

As you can see from the above, the references are limited. I am using only the reading that has triggered the key elements of this discussion. The limited reference to self-directed study in the literature means that a traditional academic approach is not feasible. It would be impossible to reference all of the material used in this chapter, as it is the result of many years of working, reading and experiencing nursing and educational practice. Sometimes it is impossible to identify which are one's own ideas and which are those of others, so I apologise for any ideas that have been shared with me (either published or simply discussed verbally), included here and not sourced.

Working out your own self-directed study journey

Now that I have identified the key themes, I shall try to explain the learning journey I take for delivering a new module written by someone else. For me, all my planned learning journeys start and finish with practice. So whether I am writing a module or a teaching plan, or interpreting module aims and outcomes, I start with the question *'What are the links to or with practice?'* Writing a new module or programme yourself is a similar journey, except that the scope of thinking is wider.

While I was working on this chapter, several groups of learners were asked to identify what they did at the start of a new module. Figure 13.1 identifies student activities at the start of a module, while Table 13.1 shows my order of self-directed study activities when preparing to deliver a module that has been written by someone else.

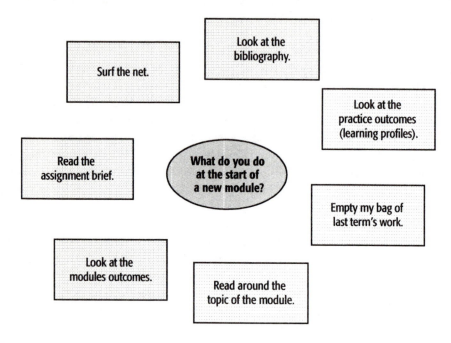

Figure 13.1 Student-identified activities at the start of a module

Perhaps completing your slant on what you do at the start of a module for study or teaching purposes might help you to identify your own self-directed study strategy. This may then enable you to guide students to their appropriate strategy, rather than impose your own or someone else's tried and tested personal route.

TABLE 13.1 Self-directed order of study for delivery of a module that has not been written by myself

Module structure	Order of activity	My self-directed learning strategy/actions	Consequences
Title	1	How does this relate to my practice and that of students?	Do I feel that this module is within my scope of expertise?
Rationale	1	What is the fit with my experience of practice (nursing, education, life, etc.)	Is this congruent with the way I think of or about education or nursing?
Aims		Where does the module fit in the programme?	

Module structure	Order of activity	My self-directed learning strategy/actions	Consequences
Learning outcomes/ objectives	2	Which of these make sense to me theoretically and practically? Literature review with my key words Discussion with colleagues	What do I know I don't know?
Content	3	Literature review with content key words	What does my new reading tell me I don't know? What is the practice I now need to explore and discuss with experts?
Put the work away for a time before planning sessions, etc. Serious thinking time!			
Assessment	4	How would I answer this? What is essential learning?	What scenarios illustrate the module? Can I analyse practice appropriately with the concepts of the module?
Practice outcomes (occasionally)	1 or 6	What competencies and clinical decisions relate to this learning?	How does my learning fit the real world? Do I view practice any differently? Is there anything that I will now change?

On reflection, my learning journey now appears structured, but this is the result of many years working in education and studying, both for myself and in order to meet work requirements. The writing of this chapter has provided the impetus to describe in words what I do as a work process. My experience with students tells me that each student approaches their work in an individual way. *It is not for me to impose my way upon them, but rather I should be helping them to work through the strengths and weaknesses of their own self-directed study, to enable them to become safe, competent and dynamic practitioners.* If you agree with this statement, the following question becomes important. How do I help a student to learn by using and developing their own self-directed learning strategies? Some cross-reference is needed here to learning styles, learning strategies and teaching styles, and I would suggest that you read the relevant chapters of books that discuss these issues in more depth (you can start by reading Chapter 1 in this book, for example).

Using the above discussion as a starting point for analysis – *working out what I need to think about next* – I shall now explore each of the identified themes from the potential perspective of learners. In addition, Table 13.2 shows one approach to an analysis of the themes with related concepts.

Table 13.2 is my strategy for working out the next lines of discussion in this chapter. The column in bold was the first one I completed, partly because it was easiest, but also because it follows my personal pattern of study (i.e. what does it mean or how does something relate to reality/practice?). The next columns were

TABLE 13.2 My stream of consciousness in respect to students' driving forces to study

Timescale	Type of targets	Theory	Tacit knowledge	Learning resources
Length of a shift or placement	Daily/hourly patient targets while in placement	Which theory should be used to explain practice – current theory being taught (keeping to curriculum design) or theory that most enables the learner to explain and understand evidence observed in practice?[11]	Each lecturer will have their own tacit knowledge that influences delivery of 'theory'	What drives structure of teaching sessions, tutorial discussions and guidance issued to students? What is essential reading?
Several weeks	Assignment deadlines	Which theory and analysis of practice is essential to pass the current assignments? Which learning may be 'lost' by energy focused on assignment achievement?	Tacit knowledge of each practitioner worked with, which influences use of 'theory' in practice	What is the appropriate activity or module design for reducing the theory–practice (tacit knowledge) gap?
1, 2 or 3 years, or more	Personal learning targets	What drives curriculum design – theory, research, tacit knowledge or evidence-based practice?[12,13]	What drives thinking – curriculum design, theory, research, tacit knowledge, evidence-based practice or life experiences?	No answers at present!!
Ongoing	Family member targets	Much research demonstrates the conflicts between home and workplace targets. Highlighted even more when reacted to the stress of achieving success in an educational/training programme.[9,14,15]	How does the tacit knowledge of everyday living conflict with or support the programme learning?	No answers at present!!
Ongoing	Cohort targets	See literature related to group dynamics and social learning theory	Tacit knowledge tells me that cohort dynamics can be crucial to learner success	Can cohort identity and cohesion affect the self-directed study of group members?
Ongoing	Site/university/QAA targets	Beyond the scope of this chapter!!		

worked out on the basis of my perspectives and understanding. This developed into the conclusions for this chapter, which raise more questions than answers.

Thinking and discussion time to help to connect theory and practice

Students and mentors are expected to work together to achieve client/patient outcomes and enable the learner to make sense of the theory that they are currently studying. Given that any of the theory, from the whole of the programme for pre-registration students, *could* be used to explain the practice observed and participated in, what should a mentor do to explain events? Should they use the most relevant theory or that which relates to current learning targets? And what happens when tacit knowledge is in conflict with conventional wisdom? The student is in the middle of a tussle between perceived wisdom and that which has not yet been fully explained. This can lead to confusion for the student and a loss of self-confidence for the mentor, who may feel that they do not know enough to teach the student. This last point is evidenced by my originally tacit knowledge but now surfacing perceptions, as a result of reviewing the current problems that mentors have in practice. My source for this knowledge is many years of teaching mentoring and assessing modules.

What happens when a student tries to put classroom learning into practice and the mentor does not perceive the relevance of this? (This scenario arose from a discussion with a mentor.) *The result is that the client/patient targets take precedence over self-directed study, which has to wait. This may be in conflict with the student's learning style.*

From the students' perspective there is potential dissonance between theory taught, tacit knowledge, as demonstrated by practitioners in placements, and the priorities of service delivery. Such conflicts can cause a reduced level of self-esteem for students. Consideration and action needs to be taken in preparation of both students and mentors to reduce the conflict by making the dissonance overt rather than covert.

Assignment deadlines

It is not disputed that assessment is necessary for successful completion of learning programmes, if for no other reason than ensuring that the newly qualified practitioner is safe to practise in professional situations. But what should be assessed? Staged points of learning or the final result? What happens when the student's understanding of practice is best served by theory other than that which is currently being taught and assessed? In an ideal world, learning – both in theory and practice – would be controlled so that the building blocks of the wall are placed in order, but practice experience cannot be controlled in this way (e.g. the student who is learning how to communicate with a patient is allowed to ignore taking a patient to the toilet because that was last term's work!).

That was a superficial example, I know, but I hope it makes the point that when the learning environment is the real world of work, any theoretical concepts may be relevant for teaching in practice. This means that students are being exposed to more than the allocated learning effort in the nice neat equation of 15 credits being equivalent to 150 hours of student effort. *The result is potential for overload as the learner tries to focus on assignment targets and associated learning, but is 'sidetracked' by the wider learning required to understand practice and follow their own self-directed study paths.*

Family member targets

Potential professionals are also members of families, with their own responsibilities and needs. Student files are littered with the evidence of constant conflict between the students' personal objectives and the requirements of the programme of study. For any student to succeed, self-knowledge of their personal strategy for self-directed study will be essential. In the first instance this allows a realisation of the time and effort that are going to be required to complete the programme. They then need to develop the strategies for lifelong learning necessary for today's professional. *The result is constant conflict between family and learning.*

Cohort targets

Many management programmes have utilised internal competition between groups to assist the learning process. Some competition is seen as a useful tool for motivating students to improve the effort that they put into the learning process. However, cohorts of students have different personalities – some foster active learning, and some cohort dynamics can actually be destructive to the learning process. The attitude of the group can either support an individual student's self-directed study or hinder it. Is the student whose classroom contribution is based on much personal study effort seen as a 'swot' or a helpful cohort resource? Are they used to reduce the study effort made by other less able or lazier students? *The result is that cohort dynamics and objectives can be either helpful or a hindrance to learners' self-directed study strategies. Teachers need to develop insight into these dynamics in order to enable cohort behaviour to work for both the individual and the cohort as a whole.*

Site/university/QAA targets and subject benchmarks

Quality assurance processes in higher education mean that the progress of students should be monitored against agreed targets (e.g. formative and summative assessments). Jackson argues that 'it is neither desirable nor possible to achieve uniform standards across the whole HE system', and consequently the 'what' and 'how' of learning must become more explicit. This reinforces the need for formative and summative assessment in ever increasing quantity, and more detailed explanation of the content of learning for professions, together with overt discussion of activities in practice. However, this is set to further burden students with content- and outcome-driven rather than process-driven education. The latter is essential for the development of a lifelong learner who is fully aware of his or her own self-directed study strategies. Quality assurance mechanisms can work against independent approaches to study and a traditional 'reading' of a subject, rather than meeting specific learning outcomes. Learners' targets of learning may therefore be devalued.

Finally, what have I learned by completing this work? Self-directed study is a complex activity which can be learned but not copied. I have found myself relating to and thinking about everything I have learned, and taught, with regard to learning, teaching and assessment within the context of professional practice. So this chapter has taken me more time than a traditional 3000-word assignment. It is the result of reading, thinking, and working in nursing and education for a considerable period of time. It makes me respect even more those practitioners who write with relevant, applicable and cogent arguments – works which students and practitioners find useful in everyday practice.

As an endnote, for those who pay attention to detail, items 5, 6 and 8 are missing from my own study topics. These were self-directed learning, study skills and work/ life balance, and reasons for choosing the named profession, respectively.

References*

* Editor's note: the author of this chapter has requested that these references be presented in the date order in which they were read, in order to maintain the themes contained within the chapter.

	Date originally read
1 QAA website; qaa.ac.uk	2000 onwards, regular review
2 College/University guidance notes.	1989 onwards
3 Evensen D, editor. *Problem-Based Learning*. London: Lawrence Erlbaum Associates; 2000.	2002
4 Eraut M. Non-formal learning and tacit knowledge in professional work. *Br J Ed Psychol*. 2000; **70:** 113–36.	2003
5 Appleton L. Examination of the impact of information skills training on academic work of health studies students: a single case study. *Health Inform Libraries J*. 2005; **22:** 164–72.	2005
6 Ottewill R. Student self-managed learning – cause for concern? *On the Horizon – The Strategic Planning Resource for Educational Professionals*. 2002; **10:** 12–16.	2003
7 Matthews P. Workplace learning: developing an holistic model. *Learn Organisation*. 1999; **12:** 272–85.	1999
8 Mezirow J. A critical theory of adult learning and education. *Adult Educ*. 1981; **32:** 3–24.	1983
9 Mezirow J. Perspective transformation. *Adult Educ*. 1978; **27:** 100–10.	1984
10 Mowrer R, Klein SB. *Handbook of Contemporary Learning Theories*. London: Lawrence Erlbaum Associates; 2001.	2005

11 Woll S. *Everyday Thinking, Memory, Reasoning and Judgement in the Real World.* London: Lawrence Erlbaum Associates; 2002.   2003

12 Wood BJG, Tapsall SM, Soutar G. Borderless education: some implications for management. *Int J Educ Manag.* 2005; **19**: 428–36.   2005

13 Eraut M. The many meanings of theory and practice (editorial). *Learn Health Soc Care.* 2003; **2**: 61–5.   2005

14 Bloomfield, Harris P, Hughes C. What do students want? The type of learning activities preferred by final-year medical students. *Med Educ.* 2003; **37**: 110–18.   2003

15 Billett S. Guided learning at work. *J Workplace Learn.* 2000; **12**: 272–85.   2001

CHAPTER 14

Applying strategies to practice

Jan Woodhouse

Introduction

There are many books dedicated to learning in practice, so this chapter cannot hope to address all the aspects that need to be considered when teaching in practice. However, it would be extremely remiss to assume that healthcare professionals learn exclusively in the classroom – students need to carry forward the ideas and theories that have been discussed and compare them with the practical setting. Likewise, practice becomes a prompt for further learning, and students will come back into the classroom and quickly compare placement experiences. Discrepancies between what their lecturer has told them and what they have witnessed in reality become

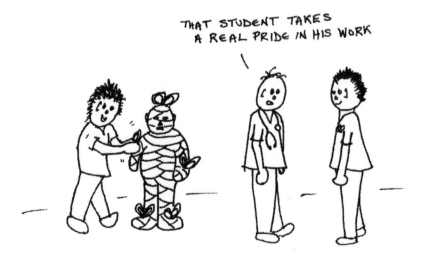

hot topics. The classroom and the practice area are symbiotic – they feed, and need, each other.

The aim of this chapter is to consider how the different teaching strategies identified in the preceding chapters can be utilised in the practice environment. I wish to thank my colleague, Liz Sweet (author of Chapter 13), for the following approach. She kindly showed me her work, in which she uses the strategies outlined by Reece and Walker[1] and considers their application in practice. The following discussion will be supported by observations drawn from years of experience of teaching at the bedside, and through many discussions with practitioners. So each strategy will be examined in terms of the advantages and disadvantage that it offers to practice. However, before we get to that point, there are a number of questions to consider. These are often remembered as '5 Ws and an H' (someone once illustrated this for me as five bottoms sitting on the cross-bar of a rugby post – try drawing it and you'll see what I mean!)

- *Who* is gaining the learning? Is it a student, a colleague, a patient or a carer? This needs to borne in mind, as consideration will then follow as to the level of prior knowledge, the language used and the relevance of the topic.
- *What* is being taught? Is it intentional or unintentional learning? The latter aspect recognises that critical incidents, near misses and bad practice can be just as informative and meaningful as intentional learning.
- *Why* is the learning happening? Is it to meet practice outcomes, to promote health education or in response to self-direction? Students may not be able to recognise the 'why' aspect. For example, I teach the concept of evidence-based practice to pre-registration nursing students and they find it difficult, at first, to see its relevance to practice.
- *When* – is it timely? Practice education is often opportunistic, and can maximise learning as everything is in context – the theory and practice come together. However, there are times when the learning comes too early – for example, when the student has not had the theory behind the practice and they may not understand what they are doing. On the other hand, learning may come too late – for example, the student may have already established a pattern of practice, and this means that they may have to relearn. Another aspect of time is the question of how much time we have to dedicate to teaching when we are in practice. The literature refers to 'micro-teaching', which recognises that we may only have 5 or 10 minutes in terms of the whole teaching process (preparation, aims and objectives, teaching strategy, assessment and evaluation). In an ideal world, time would be set aside for this process, but in reality the needs of healthcare practice can interrupt, or completely overwhelm, the teaching (and learning) process.
- *Where* – what is the learning environment like? Is it in the middle of a busy ward, a side room or a dedicated space? Are there resources available such as paper, pens, Internet access, books or journals? Most of the teaching that I have done in practice has taken place in the clinical room, at the bedside or in an empty side room with students/colleagues perched on the bed, footstools and the occasional

chair. For community staff I am informed that sitting in a car substitutes for the classroom.

- *How* are we going to teach? (The pedantic among you may ask where is 'which'? However, 'how' encompasses the 'which' aspects.) So we come to the teaching strategies. Consideration of the teaching strategy may also require you to think about the equipment you might need for that particular strategy, as well as the preceding aspects. Therefore your choice of teaching strategy will be shaped by who you are teaching, what you are teaching, why you are teaching it, when you are teaching and where the teaching takes place.

There will be times when the teaching and learning process will be incomplete, and that may feel frustrating for the teacher and the student, but this is the nature of the beast that is practice. However, it is also true that those opportunities will arise again, allowing the jigsaw pieces of knowledge to be put in place, resulting in a completed picture.

Lecture

The assumption that is made here is that information, or knowledge, flows in one direction, from the lecturer to the student. In practice, a lecture may be as short as 5 minutes. One could also include a demonstration within this category, because of the direction of the information flow.

One of the main issues to consider is where the delivery of the lecture and/or demonstration is taking place. If it is on a ward round, there may be problems with regard to confidentiality, unintended learning by bystanders and abuse of power. Space might also be a significant factor, and I have often seen a multi-disciplinary class crowding into a room in a way that would contravene any Health and Safety or fire regulations.

Advantages	Disadvantages
■ Quick transmission of information ■ Useful prior to carrying out a procedure, as it orientates the learner to the topic ■ Builds on theory and previous knowledge ■ Opportunity for other disciplines to share information ■ Maximises opportunistic learning ■ Can be delivered to varying numbers of students	■ Favours auditory learners (if a lecture) and visual learners (if a demonstration) ■ May be overheard by eavesdroppers, so consideration needs to be given to the environment in which it is given ■ Lecture can be 'hijacked' by other knowledgeable staff, which can leave the student confused if opinions differ ■ Little or no time to prepare ■ Student may not have note-taking facilities

Small groups

A small group could be regarded as a number of students in a practice setting, which could be only two students but might be more. The activity of small group learning is more likely to occur in an informal setting, such as the staff dining room, through the use of informal conversations. Consequently, the learning outcomes might be unpredictable.

The principle of keeping students 'on task' applies in practice just as it does in the classroom, so constant monitoring of the students' activity is required, otherwise you end up with students standing around waiting for the next task to be assigned to them.

Advantages	Disadvantages
■ Low numbers are less intrusive on patient care activities ■ Provides peer support for students – often called 'buddying' ■ Enhances self-directed learning ■ Students can be set tasks and given time frames for completion	■ If group size reaches five or six this can impact on patient care ■ Students may place additional demands on practice staff ■ Students might outnumber trained staff ■ Time has to be set aside for feedback on assigned tasks

Problem-based learning

This is often central to learning in practice. Problems are constantly emerging in practice, but the features of true problem-based learning, such as identifying aspects for investigation, research, facilitation of feedback and discussion, may be difficult to achieve.

In the classroom setting, students can divide up the research aspects, but in practice the task may be given to a single individual. However, this usually results in the individual becoming the local 'expert', as for example in link nurse roles.

Advantages	Disadvantages
■ Based on reality, not hypothetical ■ Encourages independent, self-directed learning	■ Requires access to learning resources ■ Requires time for feedback

Case study

Ample opportunities exist in practice for this strategy. Reading case notes and talking to patients have traditionally been practice-based activities. However, the other aspect of the case study strategy is a discussion based on directed questions. So without the questions, reading notes and discussions with patients may not be turned into a meaningful learning experience.

Therefore if you observe a student taking part in case-note reading or conversation with patients, you should consider the need to follow up their activity with a question-and-answer session.

Advantages	Disadvantages
<ul><li>Easy access to different case studies</li><li>Easy access to patients</li><li>Problems are real</li><li>Opportunity to gain multi-professional perspectives</li></ul>	<ul><li>If not facilitated, learning may not be measurable</li><li>Need time to talk to patients</li><li>May be seen as a 'time-occupying' exercise rather than a learning activity</li></ul>

Reflection

This is high on the agenda in healthcare education, whether you are in the classroom or in practice, but as Chapter 6 demonstrates, the process may not actually take place. We may have to learn how to be reflective.

So, as with case study, it is important for the teacher to facilitate reflection through the use of directed questions. This means taking the student to one side and asking about the event, what they learned, what was difficult, what they would do again, what they would do differently, and how they feel.

Advantages	Disadvantages
<ul><li>Doesn't cost anything, as it is a process</li><li>Ample experiences to reflect on</li><li>Promotes deep learning</li><li>Encourages continuing professional development</li></ul>	<ul><li>No time to discuss an experience</li><li>Mentors/teachers may not be aware of the processes involved</li><li>Tendency to focus on negative experiences rather than positive ones</li></ul>

Storytelling

In the practice setting this will normally follow the oral tradition. It is used informally and naturalistically. Stories, or narratives, may be obtained from patients – for example, their journey into illness and the effect it has had on them – or they may be passed on from colleagues.

Stories are easily identifiable because they usually start with the question 'Have you heard about . . .?' The difficulty lies in establishing whether the story is worth repeating, and to what end. Is it mere gossip or does it have a deeper meaning? If the story is worth writing down then I would suggest that it has developed meaning.

Advantages	Disadvantages
<ul><li>Enhances professional identity</li><li>Identifies archetypes – the demon doctor, the uncaring nurse, etc.</li><li>Highlights professional issues</li><li>Responsive to events</li><li>Narratives can highlight different processes at work</li></ul>	<ul><li>Unstructured, stories change with each new telling</li><li>May be regarded as 'tale-telling' or gossip</li><li>May be interrupted by other activities</li><li>Not given recognition as a teaching strategy</li></ul>

Role play

There is limited opportunity for role play as a strategy. However, role modelling is an active and subconscious activity. So in practice the student is an observer of behaviours, with the roles of practitioners being acted out in real life. Consequently, students will be exposed to all kinds of roles and situations, where both the good and the bad aspects are witnessed.

It is to be hoped that students will only pick up on the good aspects, but they cannot fail to notice the bad ones. It is important that all practitioners are made aware of their responsibilities and the impact that they can have on those around them

Advantages	Disadvantages
■ Real-life situations to observe ■ Opportunity to adopt similar behaviours ■ Student will remember good role models	■ Bad practice may be observed ■ Constant process, therefore no control over learning outcomes ■ All practitioners are involved in the process, not just the teacher

Creative activities

One does not readily associate creative activities with practice, but if you take a look around a practice area you will be hard pressed not to find some results of such activity. You will notice posters, pictures, photographs, information leaflets and the like dotted around the place. We have caught on to the idea that 'one picture is worth a thousand words.'

Usually a creative activity happens in the moment – for example, drawing a diagram to explain an operation. A drawing only needs paper and a pen, so its cost is minimal. However, you might want to produce a health education poster, in which case you would need a few more resources.

Advantages	Disadvantages
■ Allows for a different level of thinking ■ Pictorial images may aid the retention of information ■ Activity can be focused towards the needs of the client group (e.g. health education) ■ Usually low cost	■ Not regarded as 'proper' learning ■ Time and resources are needed if posters, photographs, etc. are required ■ Issues of consent arise if photographs are required

Simulation

Opportunities for the use of simulation in practice are heavily reliant on having the necessary equipment and environment. Although high-fidelity simulation equipment may not be available, you have the real thing in practice. It may be that you can practise using the equipment on a colleague instead of a patient – for example, using a slit-lamp or operating microscope.

Alternatively, you may find some low-tech equipment with which to practise. Examples that I have encountered include practising injections on an orange, and suturing gauze swabs together and practising plaster of Paris and bandaging techniques on a teddy bear.

Advantages	Disadvantages
■ The time between practice and reality is shortened	■ Problem of storage and access to equipment
■ Opportunity to observe reality before and after practising skills	■ Limited availability
	■ Reality is always different to simulation
■ Improves psychomotor skills	■ Resource implications (items such as plaster of Paris are not reusable)
■ Students can take their time when learning a skill	■ Equipment may become damaged

Experiential learning exercises

Again, opportunities abound in practice. It is important to consider the processes that are involved (i.e. identification of the emotional responses to the exercise and discussion/debriefing after the exercise). Experiential learning can range from a simple exercise, such as lying on a trolley and being wheeled through the corridors to theatre, to one that lasts a little longer – for example, having your arm in plaster for the morning.

To outsiders it may seem that those involved are just larking around, so it is important that the lead is someone who is in a position of authority, who takes time to explain to the onlookers that the activity has a purpose.

Advantages	Disadvantages
■ Helps to give understanding from a service user perspective	■ May be misinterpreted by onlookers
■ Addresses the affective domain	■ May result in negative emotions
■ Can be fun	■ Needs time for debriefing
■ Involves active participation	

Blended learning

This requires access to a computer and the Internet, which may be an issue for the employer in terms of resources. The availability of time to access the computer may also be a problem. As only one person can work on a computer at a time, the learning experience becomes an individual event.

However, the important point here is to encourage the development of an environment in which the learning can be shared and discussed. For example, colleagues may stand at your shoulder as you compose a response to a discussion thread. Alternatively, if they have composed something, they may ask you to read it through to see whether it makes sense.

Advantages	Disadvantages
■ Remains within the workplace ■ Promotes individual learning ■ Learning takes place at the student's own pace ■ Can be shared with colleagues	■ Access to resources may be a problem ■ Time is needed in which to carry out activities ■ The group may resent individual learning

Self-directed learning

Opportunity for self-directed learning abounds in practice. It is the aim of the educator to turn the student into a self-directed learner. As has been pointed out, there is an individualistic approach to self-directed learning. Some students may want to rush to complete an assignment, while others may want to take part in a concrete experience before they feel that their learning is adequate.

However, once the student has qualified, the only subsequent measure of self-directed learning will be during the annual appraisal process. Those in practice must endeavour to support the self-directed learner, for not to do so could result in lack of motivation and lowering of morale.

Advantages	Disadvantages
■ Able to identify learning opportunities ■ Able to plan own development ■ Motivational both for student and for others ■ Information flows from student to teacher	■ Seen by others as individualistic (e.g. the learner might be perceived as selfish) ■ Can cause a power imbalance ■ Does the student know what they don't know? ■ Student may not use self-directed time for study activities

Conclusion

You and others may be able to identify other examples, advantages and disadvantages of the above strategies. Practitioners often use the term '. . . if only' when talking about teaching in practice – for example, 'If only we had enough time . . .', 'If only we had the space . . .', 'If only the students came prepared . . .', and so on. This shows that the learning environment is not ideal, but it is where the application of the students' knowledge takes place. So, for all its imperfections, it is the place where the students want to be, where they learn their craft and where they try out the theory.

We started our journey, at the beginning of the book, in education at the start of the twentieth century, and here at the end we are reminded of our purpose. Our reason for being is to educate practitioners for the healthcare environment of the twenty-first century. It is an environment that is constantly changing – in fact I heard a colleague remark recently that the only thing that doesn't change in the National Health Service is the fact that it will change. It is hoped that the strategies discussed in this book will go some way towards enhancing the future education of healthcare professionals.

Reference

1 Reece I, Walker S. *Teaching, Training and Learning: a practical guide incorporating FENTO standards.* 5th ed. Sunderland: Business Education Publishers Ltd; 2003.

Epilogue

Jan Woodhouse

The writing and editing of this book have involved an interesting journey. Relationships have been strengthened, stress has (occasionally) been high, and life has carried on. Our thoughts have turned to the past, as we considered our experiences at school and during our education in the healthcare profession. The level of reflection has brought a deeper meaning to and understanding of the processes – not only those that we witness in our students in our day-to-day activities, but also at a personal level.

I realise that not every strategy which is used in healthcare education has been encompassed within the chapters of this book. For example, action-learning sets are currently being used at undergraduate and postgraduate level. The use of video recording is increasingly being used to aid communication skills. Similarly, 'sculpting' is another strategy that is used to facilitate communication skills – it is essentially role play, but here the audience supply the words to 'actors.' There is little written in the healthcare literature about these more recent and innovative teaching strategies. They haven't been fully evaluated yet, so although they may seem attractive options and alternatives to other methods, they are still in the testing phase. This means that I cannot offer them as strategies for evidence-based teaching. However, being the self-directed learner that you surely are, you might want to research them for yourself!

Writing about the past inevitably makes one consider the future, and although the subtitle of this book, *How to Teach in the 21st Century*, may seem a little presumptuous (after all, we have only just finished clearing up after the millennium celebrations), it is an opportunity to do a bit of crystal ball gazing. The rise of technology is at the forefront of change. Already I have had students arriving with laptop computers on which to take down their notes. Others seem very involved in text messages (although that isn't what they are supposed to be doing!), so it's only a matter of time before students make use of the electronic wizardry that is increasingly available and affordable. E-learning means that we don't even have to see our students. However, we cannot ignore the learning opportunity that being in a group offers, so I cannot yet envisage that we will all be able to work from home. The classroom is still necessary, and will continue to be so.

Even in the classroom, at the delivery end, the technology is developing apace and I can now move seamlessly between a PowerPoint presentation and the use of music, a video or a DVD to enhance the learning experience, whereas even a year ago I would have been slaving over a hot photocopier with a pile of acetates in my hand. It all makes for exciting times, and it would be interesting to be around at the end of the twenty-first century to see what new strategies have emerged and what current strategies have survived.

Index